REVERSING HEART DISEASE

The National Heart and Diabetes Treatment Institute regularly publishes a newsletter that updates the recent studies in nutrition as they relate to health. If you are interested in this newsletter, simply write to The National Heart and Diabetes Treatment Institute, Inc., 18800 Florida Street, Huntington Beach, California 92648. We will gladly send you an issue of the newsletter and further information about this publication.

REVERSING HEART DISEASE

JULIAN M. WHITAKER, M.D.
Introduction by Henry D. McIntosh, M.D.

WARNER BOOKS

A Warner Communications Company

Warner Books, Inc., 666 Fifth Avenue, New York. NY 10103
A Warner Communications Company

Printed in the United States of America
First Printing: June 1985
10 9 8 7 6 5 4

Book design: H. Roberts Design

Library of Congress Cataloging in Publication Data

Whitaker, Julian.
Reversing heart disease.

Bibliography: p.
Includes index.
1. Heart—Diseases—Diet therapy. 2. Low-fat diet. 3. Coronary heart disease—Prevention. 4. Aortocoronary bypass. I. Title. [DNLM: 1. Coronary Disease—diet therapy—popular works. 2. Coronary Disease—prevention & control—popular works. WG 113 W577r]
RC684.D5W47 1985 616.1'2 85-7163
ISBN 0-446-51298-2

DEDICATION

I now would like to dedicate this book to any and all individuals who read it, use it, and in any way, shape, or form benefit by that experience.

ACKNOWLEDGMENTS

It should be obvious to the reader that this book could not have been written without the enormous contribution of hundreds of scientists who have published thousands of pages of research on our most serious disease. Often, extremely important and helpful information published by insightful and intelligent researchers fails to have an impact upon clinical medicine if it runs counter to the prevailing beliefs and practices. It would be impossible for me to cite each individual who has contributed so much of the information contained in this book, but rest assured they have my undying respect and admiration for their contributions.

Closer to home I want to acknowledge Barbara Zirge and Susan Underwood, who drew upon their experience and expertise with food preparation as chefs here at the institute to compile the recipes and menu plans, which make up the most important part of this work. Without this practical information, this book would be of limited use to the reader. Sylvia Sellini, Lea Margolis, and Diana McVey were invaluable in assisting with the typing, retyping, and retyping of the manuscript. Their uncomplaining patience is greatly appreciated. A special thanks is due to Dr. Henry McIntosh for pointing out errors of commission and omission that would have hampered the purpose of this book. His editorial input was invaluable.

In addition, my editors, Bernie Shir-Cliff and Marge Schwartz, have been extremely patient, tolerant, and helpful with the multiple revisions.

And last but not least, I owe a firm debt of gratitude to patients who have completed our institute's program and have gone on to validate many of the principles outlined in this book by dramatically improving their health and enhancing the quality of their lives. Only they can take credit for that, and their experience certainly motivated me to complete this work.

"An extremely complex and costly technology for the management of coronary heart disease has evolved, involving specialized ambulances and hospital units, all kinds of electronic gadgetry and whole platoons of new professional personnel to deal with the end results of coronary thrombosis. Almost everything offered today for the treatment of heart disease is at this level of technology, with the transplanted and artificial hearts as ultimate examples. When enough has been learned for us to know what really goes wrong in heart disease, we ought to be in a position to figure out ways to prevent or reverse the process; and when this happens, the current elaborate technology will be set to one side."

Dr. Lewis Thomas

"Unless the doctors of today become the dieticians of tomorrow, the dieticians of today will become the doctors of tomorrow."

Alexis Carrel

"The doctor of the future will give no medicine, but will interest his patient in the care of the human frame, in diet, and in the cause and prevention of disease."

Thomas A. Edison

CONTENTS

DISCLAIMER

If you have a history of heart illness or believe you are a candidate for heart illness, the advice in this book can be a valuable addition to your doctor's advice, and is designed for your use under his care and direction.

INTRODUCTION

As Dr. Whitaker has emphasized coronary artery disease is the major cause of death in young and middle-aged productive individuals in this and other affluent societies of the world. But it was not always so. The frequency of coronary artery disease as the primary cause of death increased from the turn-of-the-century to about 1955. By then, it was by all odds the most important cause of death in this country—and it continues to be. Then a strange thing happened. Coronary artery disease gradually became less commonly implicated as a cause of premature death. At first, the reason for the decline was not clear. But a handful of epidemiologists looking at the disease patterns in large population groups began to get leads. One such scientist was Jeremiah Stamler.[1] In 1962, he wrote, "The accumulated evidence has made it possible to formulate an integrated general theory . . . concerning the etiology and pathogenesis of this disease. The overwhelming evidence indicates that the disease is multifactorial in causation with diet as the key essential etiologic factor . . . However, diet by itself is not a sufficient cause since premature death does not develop in all persons habitually ingesting the implicated diet." If this hypothesis was correct, it might be concluded that if there was to be a decline in the incidence of death from coronary artery disease, there would have to be a change in the dietary habits of society. Both the hypothesis and the conclusion appear to have been correct.

[1]J. Stamler, "Cardiovascular Disease in the United States," *American Journal of Cardiology*, Vol. 10, (1962), p. 319.

The importance of prevention of atherosclerosis, the basis for coronary artery disease, was also emphasized in 1962 by Dr. Stamler. He wrote, "It has frequently been said that prevention is better than cure. However, this concept has its limitations. When severe atherosclerotic disease produces organ damage, there is no cure! The statement *'prevention is better than cure'* is misleading. The public must know, policy makers and the profession must know, that the statement does not ascribe strong policy as far as atherosclerosis is concerned. They must understand precisely why prevention is essential and vital. FOR THIS DISEASE THERE IS NO CURE!" Both pronouncements by Dr. Stamler have over the years become generally accepted. And over the years, as Dr. Whitaker has indicated, although still the major cause of death, there has continued to be a decline in the incidence of death from coronary artery disease.

It has been accepted that because of this decline in the incidence of death that 630,000 persons lived in this country during the years 1968 to 1976 who would have otherwise died. Goldman and Cook,[2] based on an extensive review of the literature, concluded that this group of people lived because of the following reasons:

1. Medical interventions

Coronary Care Units	13.0%
Prehospital resuscitation	4.0%
Coronary bypass surgery	3.5%
Medical treatment of ischemic heart disease	10.5%
Treatment of hypertension	8.5%
TOTAL:	39.5%

2. Change in life-style

Reduction in serum cholesterol	30.0%
Reduction in cigarette smoking	24.0%
TOTAL:	54.0%

3. Unexplained 6.5%

TOTAL: 100.0%

[2]L. Goldman and E. F. Cook, "The Decline in Ischemic Heart Disease Mortality Rates: An Analysis of the Comparative Effects of Medicinal Interventions and Changes in Lifestyle," *Annals of Internal Medicine,* Vol. 101 (1985), p. 825.

Hypertension is a risk that can be controlled by the patient, frequently without medication. Thus, by controlling an elevated blood pressure and attaining and maintaining an ideal cholesterol level by diet and abstaining from cigarette smoking, 62.5 percent of the deaths were prevented.

It would appear that an individual-directed, prudent life-style designed to minimize recognized cardiovascular risk factors is the best insurance against death from coronary artery and other vascular diseases. Clearly, "It is what you do, hour by hour, day by day, that largely determines the state of your health, whether you get sick, what you get sick with, and perhaps when you shall die."[3]

Such conclusions accepted by increasing members of society are gratifying because for too long, large segments of the medical profession and American public have been swept along by the belief that the prevention and cure, or at least modification, of chronic diseases were most likely possible by "high tech" and/or invasive surgical approaches. In the case of coronary artery disease, this has meant bypass surgery.

I was gratified to read in *Reversing Heart Disease* Dr. Whitaker's enthusiastic support of life-style changes in the treatment of cardiac disease and diabetes. I, like he, am concerned about the excessive—frequently in my, and also his, judgment—unnecessary if not destructive utilization of bypass surgery in the treatment of many patients with coronary artery disease. I, like he, have concluded that the scientifically supported indications for surgery are far fewer than suggested by the frequency with which the procedure is currently being utilized.

But as should not be surprising, I do not agree with all of the recommendations Dr. Whitaker makes in *Reversing Heart Disease.* I do not share his enthusiasm for the chronic use of oxygen or many of the recommended vitamins. But despite my skepticism, it would be difficult to prove that they are not useful adjuncts to good health and wellness, for I know full well that enthusiasts get results that are better than those of the skeptic—not just because of the tunnel vision that so frequently is developed by the enthusiast, but because the enthusiast realizes that "a part of the cure is to want to be cured." The enthusiast is more frequently able than the skeptic to get the patient "to want to be cured."

[3]L. Breslow, Dean, UCLA Graduate School of Public Health. Quoted in "Holistic Health: Revolution or Revitalism?" *Forbes,* October 1, 1977, p. 44.

Dr. Whitaker in writing *Reversing Heart Disease* has contributed a strong stimulus to make people "want to be cured." I believe that it should be a real service to society at large and will be used by large numbers of the medical profession.

Henry D. McIntosh, M.D.,
Distinguished F. A.C.C.,
Cardiovascular Division,
Watson Clinic,
Lakeland, Florida

FOREWORD

In the spring of 1984, Dr. William P. Castelli, medical director of the Framingham Heart Study, Framingham, Massachusetts, was interviewed by *Cardiovascular News.* He stated:

> It is a sad fact that for most heart attack victims diet alone would work, if we advocated diet in American medicine—but we don't. The average patient who comes out of a coronary unit or a cardiologist's office never gets hooked up to a diet program.

This book is designed to eliminate that deficit. Combined with close follow-up with your physician, it gives you all the information necessary to add an extremely powerful tool to the treatment of heart disease. I have been using this diet and exercise program for six years on thousands of patients and found it to be extremely helpful for almost everyone. Perhaps the following case will illustrate what I mean.

Around 1973 Gene began to take medication for high blood pressure. The drugs prescribed made his uric acid rise, so more drugs were prescribed. Unfortunately, he was not given any advice about diet, exercise, or any other measures he might take to avoid what was coming.

Gene was a builder, heavily involved in his work, who dismissed his occasional chest pains as minor annoyances until September, 1979, when they became severe and frequent. Merely walking across the living room brought them on. He was given heavy doses of Inderal, nitroglycerin tablets, and a nitroglycerin patch to wear on his chest, and he was scheduled for an angiogram. This was an x-ray that showed that three of the main arteries to his heart were severely plugged by fat and cholesterol, one of them blocked completely. His doctors recommended a bypass operation. He probably would have had the operation except that he had a cold, so his operation was postponed a few days. While he was getting over the cold a friend who had heard me lecture on diet and exercise encouraged him to phone me about certain doubts and fears he had. "Dr. Whitaker," he said, "doctors in the hospital scheduled me for a major operation on my heart like they were making an appointment for a haircut. I just felt something was wrong the way I was being rushed." I told him that due to the severity of his pain, the surgery might be necessary because a bypass operation does alleviate pain. However, here at the National Heart and Diabetes Treatment Institute, we had had considerable success relieving pain with our program of diet and exercise alone. It seemed reasonable to try gentler methods before resorting to heart surgery, which by itself does not, for the most part, prevent a heart attack, stop the progress of heart disease, or prolong life.

Gene entered the Institute with other heart patients to undergo the program of treatment that I have outlined in this book. He stayed with us for twelve days in a structured environment where he was schooled in a diet and exercise program designed to reverse heart disease. The program does not just stop heart disease or slow down its progress, but could even *reverse* it by unplugging and improving the condition of blocked and hardened arteries.

The first couple of days Gene began a slow walking program. At that point his pain was so severe that he couldn't walk the 200 yards to the track, and he was taking fifteen to twenty nitroglycerin tablets a day; but after eleven days he was walking $4\frac{1}{2}$ miles and taking only three to five nitroglycerin tablets daily. Naturally, his progress pleased him. It pleased and startled us as well! We had faith in our treatment, but we had not seen so severe a case as Gene's improve in so short a time. And his improvement continued.

Eighteen months later Gene had lost twenty-five pounds, his cholesterol level had dropped from 193 to 155, his blood pressure had stabilized, he was taking no medication, and he had not felt any chest pains in over a year. Eighteen months after leaving the Institute he returned for an exercise test and a thallium scan to show the quality of circulation of the heart muscle. Both results were completely normal.

Four years later at age sixty-nine, Gene built a home gym so that he could intensify his exercise program. At that time he was not taking any medicine, his blood pressure and weight were stable, he hadn't had a chest pain in over three years, and he had returned to his former vigorous and productive life. Since his recovery he has built a sixty-unit condominium complex while working daily on his exercise and sticking to his diet. Gene got a lot out of our program, and let me say that the credit is largely his. This is not a treatment in which the doctor "fixes" a passive patient, like a plumber fixing a stopped sink. In our treatment for heart disease the doctor guides and teaches; the patients learn the treatment and its reasoning, support each other in the early stages, and continue to live wisely, conducting their own cures. The doctor is almost entirely a teacher. The patient carries out the course of treatment.

Generally, heart disease patients go to a doctor who does something to them. The bypass operation, which is described in Chapter 3 of this book, is a perfect example of something that is done to a totally passive and almost completely uninformed patient. But bypass operations, while they relieve the symptomatic pain of heart disease, do nothing to stop its progress. As the disease progresses the patient is likely to have more pains and die of a heart attack in the end. So even in those cases where bypass operations are needed, a strict postoperative course of treatment is also needed to reverse heart disease. The operation only removes a symptom of the ailment.

If you have symptomatic heart disease there is an excellent chance that you can have the same kind of happy recovery that Gene had. If you and your doctor use the program described in this book, you may expect the following improvements:

1. All the known risk factors of heart disease will be lowered or eliminated. Your blood cholesterol level will fall an average of 20 percent, or about sixty points, with most of the reduction coming from the harmful LDL fraction (see Chapter 9).

2. Almost certainly your blood pressure will fall and you may be able to stop medication for hypertension (see Chapter 8).

3. You will probably lose weight. The average weight loss with this program is four to seven pounds a month, until your weight stabilizes close to your best weight.

4. If you follow a prescribed exercise program faithfully your physical endurance will improve (see Chapter 14).

5. Chest pains will most likely diminish or stop entirely, because the oxygen-carrying capacity of your blood will increase immediately. It is often fat that reduces the oxygen supplied by the blood, bringing on angina attacks. Reducing blood fat reduces angina pectoris in most patients and eliminates it entirely in a majority (see Chapter 6).

6. Your body will handle carbohydrates more efficiently. A high-carbohydrate diet improves the way the body utilizes insulin, which in turn reduces the tendency to develop diabetes. Or, in people who have diabetes, it reduces the need for insulin or other medications.

7. The diet will increase a group of beneficial hormones called prostaglandins that decrease inflammation and reduce the tendency to premature blood-clotting as well as other beneficial effects in the human system (see Chapter 13).

8. The low-sodium, high-potassium content of the diet will help you to eliminate excess water, reducing the need for diuretics and also reducing blood pressure (see Chapter 8).

9. You will be eating less protein and producing less of the protein-breakdown products known as blood urea nitrogen or BUN. This takes stress off the kidneys, which need not work so hard to eliminate these waste products (see Chapter 10).

10. The increased fiber content of the diet virtually eliminates constipation, if you are not already habituated to laxatives or enemas. This improvement in your intestinal functioning will help the elimination of excess cholesterol and will allow your body to absorb nutrients more slowly and efficiently.

11. You will reduce or eliminate medication for heart disease. Nearly 80 percent of patients on hypertensive medication reduce or eliminate it; between 80 and 90 percent of those on anginal medication reduce or lower it. In some cases this reduction occurs within a few weeks.

We have found that these changes take place to some extent in every patient who undertakes our program, and in certain indi-

viduals the improvement is striking, as in the case of Gene. If the benefits of this program could be obtained by taking one pill, that pill would be heralded as a miracle cure for heart disease. But of course there is no such pill—only a program of diet, exercise, and appropriate medications, a program which the patient must learn about, understand, and persevere in following.

The program works best for those who learn most about it, from every angle, so it is probably best for you to know where it originates.

I grew up as the son of a doctor and was drawn to medicine early. My father is a surgeon in Atlanta, Georgia, and my brother is a radiologist there. I showed an aptitude for the sciences in high school and at Dartmouth College, and eagerly went through the four-year medical course offered at Emory University Medical School in Atlanta. After med school I began a residency in orthopedic surgery. I had completed two and a half years of the residency program when doubts assailed me. I wasn't sure how satisfied I could be following the high technology of surgery over the long haul. Successful surgeons get their greatest gratification from the drama of surgery; often, there is little personal interaction with their patients. Was that for me? I felt a need for a more personal contact with people. And there is a great deal of inside politicking in the profession of surgery, aimed at getting hospital privileges, operating room time, and referral of patients. I was impatient with that and felt that I was entering into a hidebound life in which any new idea or creativity was discouraged—even though it might help the patient and the practice of medicine. Often, the innovative surgeon finds himself rejected by his professional peers, and the rejection takes a definite form—loss of hospital privileges and referrals. With this in mind and getting me down, I decided to take off a year or two from my residency, which I fully intended to complete.

I moved to California and began working in the emergency room of a hospital. One day a young woman came in with a sprained ankle. When I saw her I was stunned. She radiated health! Her skin glowed, her eyes sparkled, her hair looked alive. All this startled me because physicians rarely deal with healthy patients. To a doctor, health is not that marvelously vital thing but simply the absence of gross disease. People vibrating with health don't go to a doctor. People in the early, silent, hidden stages of a disease, unknown to themselves, don't go to a doctor either. They go later after a crisis has developed. Doctors rarely see the early signs of disease, and they don't learn to stop its early progress. They deal with advanced illness, not with health or health maintenance.

I asked my patient why she was so obviously full of health, and she talked to me about natural foods, vitamins, minerals, and exercise. Naturally, considering my training, I thought she was crazy, one of those health-nut faddists. Just because she was so healthy didn't mean that she wasn't a nut! However, this "health nut" gave me a book describing how vitamins and minerals had been used to treat emotional disturbances in patients of Dr. Wilbur Currier in Pasadena, just twenty-five miles away.

The next week I visited Dr. Currier. He was an ear, nose, and throat surgeon who had built a large practice, over the past twenty years, based on nutrition, exercise, and preventive medicine. I was sure I could learn from him, so I went to work in his office. I stayed with Dr. Currier for two years, all the time researching the relationship between eating habits and disease. I was astonished at how much had been published on nutrition and how little of that information was being used by physicians.

After leaving Dr. Currier I spent several years studying the work of other researchers and practitioners. I spent some time at the Longevity Institute with Mr. Nathan Pritikin and left convinced that low-fat nutrition was essential to good health care. The writings of Dr. Roger Williams at the University of Texas, Dr. Jeffrey Bland at the University of Puget Sound, and Dr. Emanuel Cheraskin at the University of Alabama convinced me that nutritional supplements were important. Dr. Kenneth Cooper of the Aerobics Institution in Texas and Dr. Terrance Cavanaugh of the Toronto Heart Institute were convincing on the value of regular aerobic exercise. More recently Dr. David Horrobin, Director of the Efamol Research Institute in London, and Dr. William Connor, Professor of Medicine, Oregon Health Services University, have taught me how important certain unsaturated fats (such as primrose oil and eicosapentaenoic acid) are to production of beneficial prostaglandins.

So that is how a budding surgeon coming from a traditional medical family turned to nutrition and exercise as a treatment for heart disease. Very likely you, as a heart patient or as a reasonable, questioning reader, will want to know how that qualifies me to treat heart disease in a "revolutionary" way, luring patients away from more established courses of treatment.

The fact is that if I had trained as a cardiologist after medical school I would not likely have learned what I now know about diet and heart disease. In four years at Emory I got heavy doses of cardiology as Emory is a leading heart disease center—but only a few hours in those four years were given to the study of nutrition. Doctors are not taught nutrition in medical school, and in specialty training, nutrition is not only ignored but even scoffed at. Cardiologists are skilled technical engineers trained extensively in elaborate diagnostic techniques and in complex treatments with drugs and surgery. The modern cardiologist, with all his high skills, is neither versed nor particularly interested in the nutritional treatment of heart disease.

Cut loose from the conventional pursuit of specialty training I was free to use the most valuable skill to be acquired in a medical education: the ability to use the medical library. This book is a product not only of my own experience in treating more than 2,000 heart patients but also of more than ten years of continued research into the latest data on nutrition and its effect on heart disease.

My work with heart patients has been exciting and fascinating because it has been working in new territory. And I could never have acquired the special knowledge or have developed the Institute treatment program we use to help patients if I had not struck out in my own direction.

Practicing medicine in this unorthodox way has its own great rewards, and not the least of these is my own improved health. I practice what I preach about diet and exercise, and this encourages my patients. Much of the time I share the same meals and—to the surprise of new patients just starting the program—enjoy them immensely. It makes teaching the program much easier. As I continue to learn about the heart and nutrition and to adjust the program to my latest findings, I feel better and function better myself, and thus learn something about good health that can be learned in no other way. Health, if considered only as the absence of disease, is not understood at all. Truly great health is experiencing life fully, having and using an abundance of energy, interest, and pleasure in your own experience of living. How you feel is the one true standard of the quality of your life. Accomplishments, money, and status are important but health is the highest reward of wise living.

As a physician I take pleasure in watching people undertake a diet and exercise program and begin to understand what a sense of well-being is all about.

Interest in diet, exercise, and health is increasing all over the country and you are no longer considered a "health nut" if you show a devotion to these things. This movement has certainly taken hold of my efforts; I am conscious of being part of a large popular movement. To avoid heart disease and to reverse heart disease you must understand the treatment because you will have to administer the treatment yourself. Hurling yourself into a diet and exercise program without guidance and information may do more harm than good.

This book is designed for use with your own physician. It provides you and your physician with what is lacking in the current therapy for heart patients—a vigorous diet designed to produce the maximum results that can be reasonably expected from nutrition. This book is not a challenge to your physician's role in your treatment; rather, it is designed to help him help you by providing you with the education needed to change your eating habits successfully. Many cardiologists are very supportive of these dietary principles, but their practices and responsibilities make it difficult for them to supply you, the patient, with the education necessary for successful dietary change. With this book, both you and your physician have the necessary tools.

This diet and exercise approach to heart disease will not put established medicine out of business, nor would any sane health authority want it to. There will continue to be progress in new drugs, diagnostic techniques, and surgery—marvelous developments when properly applied in cases where they are needed. But we must remember that all that high technology is aimed at the treatment of symptoms, not the causes of illness. We should all heed the words of Hippocrates, the father of medicine, who said:

> It appears to me necessary for every physician to be skilled in nature and to strive to know, if he would wish to perform his duties, what man is in relation to the articles of food and drink and to his other occupations, and what are the effects of each of them on everyone. Whoever does not know what effects these things produce upon man cannot know the consequences which result from them. Whoever pays no attention to these things, or paying attention to them does not comprehend them, how can he understand the diseases which

befall man? For by every one of these things a man is affected and changed this way and that, and the whole of his life is subjected to them—whether in health, convalescence, or disease. Nothing else, then, can be more important and necessary than to know these things.

PART I

The American Way to Die

1

The American Way to Die

Almost two million Americans die each year of various causes—a reasonable figure, perhaps, in a nation of well over two hundred million. But close to half are dying of one avoidable ailment, and that is too many. Nearly one million people each year die in this country of heart disease and related cardiovascular ailments, all related to bad diet, smoking, and inadequate exercise. It's the American way to die. The fellow who is killing his arteries and his heart is so common that we consider it natural! It's the way to die if you want to be an all-out contender, according to a certain school of thought. If you're living recklessly—to the hilt, working too hard, playing too hard, stuffing yourself with steaks and hamburgers (just no time to eat right), never thinking of tomorrow—then you're a prime candidate for a heart attack. The guy who courts death with heart disease in some way is unconscious and inflexible in his thinking "Meat and potatoes is a man's food, and no one can tell me differently!" This is ignorance and it is pervasive at all levels of society—even by doctors who should know better.

I recall reading a news item about a doctor who died at the wheel driving through a South Dakota blizzard to make house calls on patients who couldn't get to the hospital. He was the real thing, no doubt about it, but to me the story had a special meaning. Here was a highly educated, dedicated health professional skilled in caring for his patients who didn't know how to protect himself against the most common and most avoidable killer—heart disease.

An Artificial Tragedy

The high rate of heart disease in this country (and in most countries where a European-style diet dominates) is not a natural phenomenon, nor is it inevitable. The causes of heart disease are known and the ailment is avoidable. Furthermore, if you have heart disease, it is possible to reverse its progress and bring your arteries back to a healthier condition—not by harsh measures but by a simple, gentle natural change in life-style. Not to a less active life-style but one that is more active.

Heart disease is not a disease of the elderly. It isn't the merciful release at the end of a long life. Heart disease is killing people in the prime of life, swiftly and often without warning. It is a fatal tragedy that we read about almost daily in the newspaper.

Consider this example: He was only forty-eight and life was paying off. His career was cresting, he had just married, he had everything to live for and every intention of living for it. As far as he knew, his health was superb, but in the early morning hours of January 13, 1980, David Janssen, the star of "The Fugitive" and "Harry-O," was felled by a massive heart attack. He had no prior history of heart disease.

A million people a year dying of heart disease is not news—people take it for granted. If there is a big story about a fatal heart attack, it makes the front page in the newpapers because the person is famous, and not because there is much interest in the ailment. Dying of heart disease is as unnecessary as dying of drug abuse, yet it is taken as a normal thing. When Peter Sellers died at fifty-four the hospital spokesman said he died of "natural causes." But there is nothing *natural* about dying of heart disease at fifty-four. Heart muscle and blood vessels are meant to last a lot longer than that.

Heart disease is treacherous, and most often kills without warning. Forty-four percent of death by heart failure comes this way. Every year 400,000 people die without knowing what hit them. No warning twinges of angina give them a chance to take any steps against heart disease. Paul Lynde, famous for his quick wit on "The Hollywood Squares," didn't show up at a party. He was found dead of a heart attack at home. Congressman William Steiger of Wisconsin was felled the same way. But though sudden heart attack is common enough, it is no more *natural* than death or injury by gunshot or car accident.

I want to emphasize that heart disease kills without warning. People who have not had any symptoms of heart disease—chest pains or shortness of breath—don't realize that the process of atherosclerosis (a dangerous clogging of the arteries) takes place without pain. The fact is that if you live on the conventional American diet, fed to you since babyhood, then you can expect atherosclerosis is destroying your arteries right now.

The Well-Fed Fallacy

"Good food" to Americans means a lot of animal protein—meat, eggs, cheese, cream sauces, etc. Taken as a whole, Americans consume on the average 40 percent of their calories as fat, 20 percent as protein, and 40 percent as carbohydrates. Almost every meal conforms to this caloric composition: bacon, eggs, toast, butter, coffee, milk for breakfast, hamburger or other meat sandwich usually with mayonnaise for lunch, and a hearty dinner of steak, vegetables, bread, and salad (with a fatty dressing) for dinner.

The purpose of this book is largely to urge people off the celebrated American way of eating and dying, a difficult task, to say the least. However, I have had a great deal of success getting people to modify their habits by educating them on what to expect and why.

One reason for the difficulty in changing our eating habits is that we are conditioned to the tastes and consistency of the foods we have had since childhood. A thick juicy steak not only tastes good but is a not so subtle statement that all is "well." Even the names of the meats—prime rib, choice cut, grade A—give the American a hearty sense of well-being. I often marvel at how destructive we Americans can be with our food selection, while at the same time we actually believe we are doing ourselves a favor. This dangerous conditioning is so strong that many American men wear their obesity, high blood pressure, heart disease, and corroded arteries almost with a macho pride.

The nutritional problems of the poorer countries are those of food scarcity. Our problems, however, are those of not only too much food, but the wrong type. Our country's founders brought with them certain notions about what people just naturally wanted to eat. As we flourished, our ideas about eating became more and more a national disaster—a culturally induced mistake that has made us a nation of plugged arteries and heart attacks.

I don't expect to override all the training and brainwashing that have addicted us to our national diet, but I know I can chip away at it. This book will make some converts among people who want to avoid early death, pain, gangrene caused by stopped arteries, dangerous and traumatic surgery, invalid existences, and all that is associated with heart disease. This is a book for those of you who want to live—and to live longer and better.

What I propose for you is entirely doable. And it is not a life of deprivation—quite the opposite. When you get into this plan you'll know that you have never lived better nor as well. But before you begin you must have a certain goal in mind and a picture of a new life-style that is very desirable.

A Beautiful Mental Image

You need a beautiful mental picture of a healthy heart, lungs, arteries, and blood doing their long work as they are meant to. Keeping that positive image in your mind will encourage you to improve your health.

The blood and its constituents and functions is a lifelong study, and an entire book the length of this one would serve as no more than an introduction to the subject. For our purpose we'll consider the blood as a fluid that carries oxygen and nutrients to all the live cells of the body. The oxygen is picked up by the blood as it flows through the blood vessels of the lungs, and the nutrients are absorbed by the blood from the walls of the intestines. Since we have considerable control over what we eat and what we breathe we can do a great deal to get the right things into our blood and keep the wrong things out of it. As to what we breathe, we can fight air pollution and abstain from smoking. We have a wide choice of things to eat in our supermarkets and can easily keep ourselves supplied with healthy and delicious food.

The heart in the wisely fed body, barring any of the rather rare genetic or accidental abnormalities, works like this: the bluish blood collected from the body by the veins is taken into a chamber of the heart called the right auricle. From there it enters the right ventricle, a pumping chamber, and the contractions of the right ventricle force this de-oxygenated blood into the lungs, where it acquires a fresh load of oxygen. Now bright red again, the blood flows from the lungs into the left auricle. This chamber serves as a steady, gentle pump to keep the left ventricle supplied with arterial blood. The left ventricle in turn pumps the blood vigorously into the arterial system through the aorta, the biggest artery in the body. The powerful pumping of the left ventricle pushes the renewed blood from the aorta into all the arteries of the body. Day and night, night and day, all the long life of the human being from before birth to the last moment of life the muscle walls of the left ventricle continuously relax and contract about sixty times a minute. To keep this work up the heart needs a constant supply of bright red arterial blood which it gets straight from the aorta by way of the right and left coronary arteries.

The Coronary Arteries

These two arteries are wrapped around the exterior of the heart, branching out to carry blood to the constantly working organ. If the heart is the hardest-working organ of the body, the coronary arteries are the hardest-used arteries. They are constantly moved by the vigorous movements of the heart wall that they supply. Treated well, the hard-working coronary arteries will serve the heart for long beyond our Biblical expectation of a seventy-year life span.

These are the arteries involved in what is variously called coronary heart attacks, massive coronaries, or coronary infarctions. All those names mean the same thing: coronary arteries clogged and thus unable to deliver fresh blood to the galloping walls of the heart. When you know a little about the heart and the coronary arteries you may very well find yourself amazed in two ways. First to realize how well heart and arteries can serve for so long; and second to think that millions of people in our high-tech society have no knowledge of the simple rules that will keep their arteries and heart working well.

Fat, Oil, and Blood

Good arterial blood carrying oxygen and nutrients to all the living tissues, muscles, skin, and organs, moves most easily through the blood vessels into the tissues as a thin fluid without excess fat, oil, or cholesterol. The capillaries are wide enough only to let the blood cells through single file; cells that are clumped together by fat and oil don't get through those tiny vessels.

So thin, well-oxygenated blood serves the body best, and what it does for the other parts it also does for the heart muscle and the tissues of the arteries that carry the blood. Getting the good, freely moving blood to the cardiovascular tissues is of the utmost importance. Well-nourished and oxygenated by good blood, the blood-supplying system itself works better and lasts longer. Heart disease, to use the name applied to the most common ailment of the cardiovascular system, is actually artery disease that ultimately destroys the heart muscle. Like drug abuse, this artery disease is usually self-inflicted.

The Role of Cholesterol

Fat and oil in the blood turn it from a thin, nutritious, oxygen-bearing fluid into a heavy sludge which is harder for the heart to push through the arteries and into the smaller blood vessels. Excess cholesterol builds obstructions inside the arteries thereby narrowing them and making the heart's work harder still. I said *excess* cholesterol because a certain amount is needed by the body (see Chapter 9). How much is enough, and how much is too much? Few questions have a simpler answer. The body itself manufactures all the cholesterol it needs. Any additional cholesterol that we take in can only be harmful, and the more of it we take in the more harm it does. The cholesterol we ingest comes from animals: flesh, organ meat, milk and milk products, fish, chicken, and eggs. There is no cholesterol in any vegetable matter.

The harm done by excess cholesterol in the blood results from its attraction to already damaged cells. Some damage to the interior walls of arteries is inevitable, but the presence of fat and oil and carbon monoxide from smoking is likely to do extra damage. Without excess cholesterol the damage to the cellular lining of the arteries would mend well enough leaving small damage. But the excess cholesterol is drawn into the injuries. It intermingles with the cells of the lining, making a swelling around the injured area that continues to develop into a cholesterol plaque that can block the artery completely. These permanent lumps in the arteries continue to build as long as there is excess blood cholesterol causing the "hardening" and narrowing that makes the heart's work harder and that lessens the supply of blood to all body cells beyond the constricted point. When the supply of blood is not enough to keep body cells alive—whether they are cells in your toes or cells in your heart muscle—those cells become necrotic. Dead.

Those Heart Statistics and You

The above description is a simplified account of the process of damage to arteries and body tissues by excess blood fat and excess blood cholesterol—the process behind the statistics of death from heart attack and other cardiovascular causes. And I repeat: if you eat like a traditional American, this process is going on in your body now.

At the beginning of this chapter I said that half the people who die in the average year succumb to cardiovascular disease. Let me be less general. In 1981 there were 1,987,000 deaths resulting from all causes, and 978,360 deaths from cardiovascular disease. Deaths by accident came to 102,130; by car accident, 52,300. Deaths by homicide were no more than 24,600. The news media make a big fuss about deaths by accidents, especially car accidents, and they give a lot of play to deaths by homicide. But all of these together are small potatoes next to deaths from heart disease.

What do these numbers mean to you? Roughly, that your chance of dying of heart disease is one out of two. But whether you are learning about the likelihood of heart disease now for the first time or have already had one or more heart attacks, you can improve your chances of survival to a ripe age, improve the quality of the rest of your life, and even reverse the deterioration of your arteries. All this without surgery, and probably without heavy medication or a restricted life-style. You can do that. It's very much up to you.

Isn't Heart Disease Inherited?

For some reason there is widespread belief that heart disease is an inherited disease, with family history playing the strong role in who is to suffer and die from it. In reality, heart disease is a nutritional disease for the overwhelming majority, and family history has little to do with it. Let's examine the role of inherited traits with respect to heart disease.

It is easy to understand why this disease is thought to be inherited. With over half of the population dying from heart disease, with it killing fifty-five out of every hundred Americans, it is hard to find a family that has escaped its treachery. If one's father, uncle, grandmother, and brother all die from this disease at various ages, concern about one's own fate is automatic. However, just because heart disease is very frequent, striking many families, this does not in any way indicate, by itself, that it is inherited.

If this disease were inherited, then the incidence of this disease would be more or less constant. This is certainly the case with other inherited diseases, like mongoloidism, muscular dystrophy, hemophilia, and cystic fibrosis, all transmitted by a gene mutation and easily traceable among families. The incidence of these diseases is more or less constant from culture to culture.

Heart disease is quite different. For instance, the Japanese culture suffers very little heart disease in Japan, roughly one-tenth of that suffered in the United States. However, when the Japanese migrate to the American shores and take up the American life-style and diet, within one generation the rate of heart disease goes up tenfold, equaling what we Americans suffer. If heart disease were *primarily* an inherited disease, the protection afforded the Japanese in Japan would come with them to our shores.

True, there is the inherited tendency in a small group of individuals for extremely elevated blood cholesterol levels. These patients generally have cholesterol levels well above 300, and many of them do indeed die early from heart disease. This tendency, however, has a frequency of only 1 out of 500 in our culture and in other cultures as well. Since one out of two deaths in our culture is attributable to heart disease, then obviously this inherited tendency does not contribute significantly to the death of the overwhelming majority who die. The average cholesterol level of the American population today is about 211, and the average cholesterol level of those who suffer their first heart attack is only 220. Obviously, these are very low cholesterol levels when compared to those few individuals with the inherited tendency for cholesterol levels above 300. The cholesterol levels in the mid-200 range are the consequence of our diet and our diet alone, with inherited tendencies having little to do with it.

As all of us know, there are several factors which contribute to progressive atherosclerosis and heart disease. If this disease therefore were inherited, did these individuals inherit high blood pressure, cigarette smoking, stressful, inactive living, obesity, and the myriad of other factors known to play a part? Of course not. These are factors of culture, not genes, and unlike the genetic factors, are certainly under our control.

Even more important, the few individuals who have inherited the tendency to elevated cholesterol did not also inherit corroded arteries. Corroded arteries develop in them as a result of the elevated cholesterol, just as they develop in those of us who eat our way to atherosclerosis. Unlike patients with hemophilia, muscular dystrophy, or other truly inherited diseases, we can control the inherited tendency of elevated cholesterol levels with appropriate diet and medications. With some, the task may be difficult, but for no one is death from cardiovascular disease a foregone conclusion.

What bothers me most about our concentration on heart disease as an inherited problem is that for both doctor and patient it sets the stage for inactivity: "Oh well, it's in my genes." This attitude can be deadly and should be resisted by all. If I had my way, I would eliminate any discussion of this disease being inherited until we became expert at eliminating the risk factors in the millions who will die from it because of ignorance, poor eating habits, and dangerous living.

Stress—Isn't It a Major Factor in Heart Disease?

Rarely a day goes by without someone informing me of how important stress is in the development of heart disease. There has been so much written about stress as a factor in not only heart disease but other diseases that many believe it to be the only cause. Stress can be the straw that breaks the camel's back, bringing on the heart attack, but it is our diet and life-style which set the stage.

The role that stress actually plays is, in my opinion, overrated and misunderstood.

If we examine our foreign neighbors, we find that stress doesn't seem to play a major part in heart disease. For instance, the Japanese characteristically live in a very crowded, stressful environment. As a culture, they are extremely competitive and driven to excel, so much so that they have almost taken over many of our industries. Yet heart disease in their country is less than one-tenth of what it is in our country. When they come to the United States, however, guess what happens? As they change their diet, their heart-disease death rate increases tenfold.

Secondly, the stress upon the civilian population of Europe during both World War I and II certainly did not increase the death rate from heart disease. In fact, the death rate from heart disease fell—dramatically. This decrease resulted from a reduction in the rich, high-fat, cholesterol foods.

Even within our own culture, it is difficult to pinpoint the role that stress plays in cardiovascular disease. For instance, it is commonly believed that increasing responsibility creates additional stress that can lead to heart disease, but the studies dispute this. Dr. Lawrence E. Hinkle, Jr., head of the Division of Human Ecology, Department of Medicine and Psychiatry, Cornell University Medical College, completed a five-year perspective survey of 270,000 Bell Telephone Company employees. He wanted to see if climbing the corporate ladder leads to increased heart-attack rates as many of us believe. If so, then those in upper management levels with more responsibility and stress would be expected to have more heart attacks. This was the largest study of its time ever undertaken. At the end of the study he found no relationship whatsoever between management level and the incidence of heart attacks. According to Dr. Hinkle, the study "didn't come out the way I anticipated." There was an equal number of heart disease in blue collar and middle management personnel as in upper management personnel. Dr. Hinkle concluded that "heart disease is not greatly influenced by the tensions of adult life in an industrial society, but is related to such factors as body build, smoking, eating habits, and social and educational background, all of which are determined by the time the adult stage is reached."

Dr. Meyer Friedman indicts a personality type as a cause of

cardiovascular disease. In his book *Type A Behavior and Your Heart,* he paints the picture of an individual who is competitive, a slave to times and schedules, easily irritated and frustrated, and often, but not always, "successful" and hard driving. Many believe that this type of personality, with all its stressful characteristics, runs a greater risk of heart disease, and some list it as a definite, though minor, risk factor.

There are certain problems with this concept. First, the identification of the Type A is not clearly defined and is based on responses to a questionnaire as well as the physician's recorded observations about the patient's demeanor and conduct. Therefore, the method of testing is wide open to inaccuracy. Secondly, it is difficult to take the measurement of the "degrees" of Type A present in an individual and derive meaningful statistics about how much these factors contribute to his risk. We know clearly that even a slight reduction or increase in the blood cholesterol level is very significant in terms of risk of death, but what sort of statistical comparison can we make between the person who has only a few Type A characteristics and the person who is a definite Type B or Type A?

In spite of these obvious flaws, many physicians and even more patients seem to believe that these personality characteristics are definitely a factor. However, a recent study by Dr. Richard B. Shekelle, director of epidemiology and biostatistics in preventive medicine at Chicago's Rush–Presbyterian–St. Luke's Medical Center, found that Type A was not specifically linked to heart disease. In 1,550 middle-aged men followed for an average of seven years, those showing Type A traits wound up with no more heart attacks or cardiac events than those with Type B or more placid personalities.

Even though it is statistically difficult to relate Type A personality to cardiovascular disease, I do believe that stress and type of personality play a role in heart disease and in other diseases. I also believe, however, that the inordinate amount of discussion about stress and its effects have done us a disservice. It has deflected our attention away from diet, exercise, and other vigorous risk-factor controls that, regardless of the effects of stress, play a known and very important part in the development of heart disease. Therefore, for those individuals who are known to be Type A or who are in stressful situations, I would strongly recommend that they first and foremost get their blood cholesterol level to 160 or lower, adequately control their blood pressure and weight, and start a mild exercise program as a first priority. Then, and only then, should they concentrate on stress reduction or personality alterations. Let's put our priorities where we know we will have an effect. Indeed, I cringe every time I hear someone explain: "You know you can eat anything you want if only you could learn to control your stress."

2

Heart Disease and Modern Medicine

Without question there have been enormous advances in the tools available to the modern physician for treating patients with heart disease. In the 1950s, heart attack victims were generally treated with bed rest, watchful concern, and hope that the injured heart muscle would heal. Today, treatment is much more sophisticated: Heart attack victims are placed in special coronary care units where the heart rhythm and other functions are carefully monitored. Drugs are available that can control the heart rhythm, slow the heart, and even reduce the amount of oxygen that is required by the heart muscle. Pacemakers, now routine, can pace the heart when it is needed. Secondly, we now have the technology (the heart-lung machine) to stop the heart completely while doctors perform elaborate surgery on the heart's blood vessels (the bypass—to be discussed later), a procedure that was undreamed of in the 1950s. These advancements are believed by almost all physicians and patients to be lifesaving for thousands, perhaps hundreds of thousands of heart patients a year.

Most of the advancements now available to modern physicians, however, are tools for "managing" the problem of heart disease once it has become manifest. Even today's sophisticated diagnostic tools, such as nuclear scans and computer-assisted angiograms (special x-rays), are techniques for the early detection of heart disease so that management technology can be utilized. Very few of the tools used by the modern physician are geared toward eliminating the cause of the atherosclerotic blockage or, for that matter, even slowing down the progression of the disorder. The question arises—how lifesaving is this improved management of progressive heart disease?

Over the last fifteen years there has been a dramatic decrease in death from coronary heart disease. As Dr. Robert I. Levy of the National Heart, Lung, and Blood Institute discusses (*Atherosclerosis.* 1:312–325, Sept.–Oct., 1981) heart deaths decreased by 29 percent from 1968 to 1978. Considering that over a million people died from heart disease in 1968, a 29-percent reduction means that well over 250,000 lives are now being saved each year and the decrease in heart deaths is continuing. Is this decline the result of better medical management of victims of heart disease, or is it the result of fewer cases of heart disease in the culture, which would be primary prevention?

The Case for Better Treatment

The case for better treatment of patients of heart disease as a major reason for the declining death rate is not very strong. First, the majority of those who die from heart disease die outside of the hospital away from the benefits of modern technical intervention. An alarming number, close to half of those who succumb to heart disease, die at the first symptom of the disease and would never under any circumstances have the opportunity to benefit from the advancements of improved management.

It can be said that death in the modern coronary unit has been dramatically reduced. The ability to monitor the rhythm of the heart and alter these rhythms immediately with drugs has reduced the death rate in these specialized units from 30 to 15 percent over the last decade. But what is the fate of patients discharged from the hospital? A particularly alarming study from Johns Hopkins Medical Center by Dr. R. Goldberg (Time trends in prognosis of patients with myocardial infarction: a population-base study, *Johns Hopkins Medical Journal.* 144:73–80, 1977) indicated that the one-, two-, and three-year survival rates of patients who have suffered a heart attack is about the same as it was ten years ago.

Certain drugs called beta blockers do seem to have a beneficial long-term effect on death rates on patients who have suffered a heart attack. Studies in Europe have shown that these drugs lower the death rate of such patients, and studies published recently here in America have likewise indicated lowered death rates. As Dr. Levy points out, though, we cannot say at this time that these drugs played a major role in the overall reduction of death rate in heart disease that has occurred since 1968, because they did not become widespread until the midseventies, a time when the reduction in death was already well underway.

One of the most dramatic methods of handling heart disease is bypass surgery (to be discussed separately). With respect to this treatment, we can safely say that it has not participated in any significant way in the decline of the death rate. Even though it is currently done very frequently—over 170,000 times a year—we now know that only a small percentage of those who receive this operation have had their lives prolonged by the procedure. Secondly, considering the magnitude of the decline—250,000 lives saved each year since 1968—in order for the bypass operation to play any significant role in this reduction, it would have to save a large percentage of those undergoing the procedure rather than just a handful. Even if it saved everyone, which is an absolute impossibility, it would still account for only about 40 percent of the decline.

Given the enormous number of patients who still die from heart disease as well as the nature of this progressive disorder, one can reasonably conclude that bypass surgery and approaches similar to it (e.g., angioplasty, a technique where a balloon on the end of a catheter is used to force open plugged arteries) will most likely never play a major role in overall death rates of heart disease in this country. This does not mean that these procedures cannot be used beneficially for management of heart disease, but the declining mortality figures seem to result from factors other than the improved management techniques available for treating men and women who suffer from heart disease.

The Case for Prevention

The case for prevention is stronger—but not proven. The explanation for the declining death rate appears to be an actual decline in the disease itself. Fewer people seem to be having heart attacks; the process of atherosclerosis seems to be slowing down in the culture at large, and the disease seems to be on its way out, at least compared to the magnitude of occurrences in the past.

Dr. G. D. Friedman from the Kaiser-Permanente medical-care program in California reported a steady decline in admission for acute heart attack from 4.05 per 1,000 admissions in 1971 to 2.96 per 1,000 in 1977, a 27-percent reduction. The fatality rate for the heart attack victim did not change appreciably over that period, with 13 percent dying as a result of the attack in 1971, compared to 16 percent in 1977. This would obviously indicate that the reduction in overall death rates appears to be an actual decline in the incidence of the disease, since the death rates for those that did have a heart attack did not change appreciably, at least not at this medical center.

Sidney Pell, Ph.D., reported results of a twenty-three-year study of a large population of men working for E. I. du Pont de Nemours and Company, Wilmington, Delaware. Between 1957 and 1964, 3.13 men per 1,000 suffered a heart attack. However, from 1973 to 1979 2.57 per 1,000 suffered a heart attack, an 18-percent reduction. Interestingly, the heart attack rate dropped by 11 percent in wage employees but by 26 percent in salaried employees. Dr. Pell went on to elaborate that in other studies, the average reduction in serum cholesterol over the last twenty years has been most marked in men with at least some college education and in those with annual incomes of $10,000 or more. In his study he found that improvements in medical care, as measured by the rate of survival among men who had a myocardial infarction, probably accounted for only a small portion of this reduction in death rate. He concluded that "a reduction in the incidence of myocardial infarction, rather than an improvement in postinfarction medical care, is probably the major cause of the recent decline in myocardial infarction death rate."

I would certainly hope that the reader does not get the wrong idea. Heart disease is still the number-one cause of death and will likely remain so throughout our lifetimes. This book is designed to help you stay out of those mortality statistics. This is no time to rest on our laurels.

A careful examination of some of the changes that have occurred in the American society since 1968 seems to indicate that we, as a society, are taking the steps necessary to eradicate the disease. As will be discussed in Chapter 14, Americans are much more conscious of the benefits of physical activity. Also, Americans have made substantial reductions in their diet since the midsixties. Since 1963, fluid milk and cream consumption are down 22 percent, butter consumption down 36 percent, eggs are off 14 percent, saturated fats are down 48 percent, vegetable oils are up 74 percent. This translates into a reduction in total dietary cholesterol intake from 600 to 800 milligrams a day in the midsixties to less than 500 milligrams now. These dietary changes have resulted in a significant drop in blood cholesterol levels (see Chapter 9)—from 3 to 8 percent in each age group. According to data newly published by the Lipid Research Clinic, this drop in cholesterol level, by itself, could possibly have reduced the death rate from heart disease by as much as 16 percent. That would account for saving 160,000 lives a year from diet changes alone since the midsixties.

In addition there has been a 29-percent reduction in use of tobacco over the last fifteen years—most of this reduction by men over the age thirty, who are keenly susceptible to heart disease. This surely has played a significant role in the declining death rate of not only heart disease but also stroke death, which has fallen 40 percent since the midsixties. As you may know, stroke can result from the process of atherosclerosis just as heart disease does.

To a great extent these changes in society have, at least indirectly, been the result of medical progress and research, and of the society's education, which the medical community has supported. As pointed out by Dr. Levy in his excellent review, the cardiovascular epidemiologists claim that the calculated reduction in risk achieved by all of the life-style changes since 1968 can explain the entire decline that has occurred since that time in the death rate from cardiovascular disease.

One form of treatment that is dispensed routinely from many physicians' offices and that may have contributed to the decline of heart death has been the more aggressive control of high blood pressure. It is interesting to note that the diet changes Americans have made since the midsixties (as discussed in Chapter 8) could also be expected to reduce blood pressure. Furthermore, some of the drugs commonly used for treatment may have actually increased the death rate (see Chapter 8). Be that as it may, good blood pressure control, whether by diet or by safe drug-therapy, would be expected to contribute to the declining death rate of heart disease and, to a greater extent, of stroke.

Blood pressure control, however, is considered to be a preventive technique and represents a very small fraction of the time and effort spent by the modern cardiologist. As pointed out, most modern physicians spend the majority of their time in the technical management of the disease once it has manifested itself. In fact, many heart patients do not get from their personal physicians any information at all on appropriate dietary changes—or for that matter, any strong, effective encouragement to stop smoking. In the recent studies on the effectiveness of bypass surgery (the CASS study is discussed below), patients in both the surgical group (those who had the operation) and the medical therapy group had no significant change in their blood cholesterol levels or smoking habits over the five years of the study. This study was published in 1984, long after the time when heart specialists should have been routinely making effective changes in their patients' habits.

No one can say for sure at this point what part either primary prevention of the disease or improved care of the patient has played in the declining death rate of heart disease. Nevertheless, it is discouraging that so much emphasis and money is being spent on improving the technology for management of the disease, and not nearly enough on its causes and, thus, its prevention. It is also particularly discouraging at this date that the most expensive advancement in management—bypass surgery—has so far played no significant role in the declining death rates and is not likely to, even though the price tag for this technique is well over 2 billion dollars a year.

What is true is that there will be continued advancement in treating and managing this disease. When it comes to isolating and eliminating the cause, I do believe that the program in this book is a fast step forward. Designed to be used by you with your cardiologist, it represents, at least at one level, a wedding of primary prevention and acute management. If we as patients and physicians used both approaches simultaneously, the death rate from this dreaded disease would fall even more rapidly. As Dr. Levy concluded in his article: "The decline in the Coronary Heart Disease epidemic in the 1970s strongly suggests that we can control and even eventually eradicate modern civilized man's most serious killer disease."

3

Bypass Surgery— Pros and Cons, Risks and Benefits

The bypass operation is certainly a dramatic, expensive, and dangerous therapy for patients with heart disease. Approximately 170,000 operations are done each year at a cost of over 2 billion dollars. This procedure has become the most common operative procedure ever, outstripping the tonsillectomy and the hysterectomy in their heyday. The bypass is also the most controversial, and unlike tonsillectomies and hysterectomies, it has been surrounded by controversy from the beginning.

In spite of this, however, this operation and the technology supporting it is almost worshiped by a large number of cardiologists and surgeons. It is recommended with such confidence and enthusiasm by so many cardiologists that, from the patient's view, there seems to be neither controversy about nor alternative to its use. Because this operation does cause significant damage to everyone who receives it, very careful analysis of it as a form of therapy for heart disease is necessary.

How Did It Start?

In the midsixties two significant advancements made bypass surgery possible. First was the development of the angiogram, a special x-ray that utilizes a catheter to inject dye into the coronary arteries showing the location and severity of atherosclerotic blockages. The second was development of the heart-lung machine that takes on the function of both heart and lungs. During bypass surgery the heart must be stopped in order to sew in the grafts; the patient's blood is then pumped to the heart-lung machine, which filters out carbon dioxide, adds oxygen, and pumps the blood back into the patient's body. With the angiogram pinpointing the blockage and the ability to stop the heart for surgery, the bypass operation was born.

What Is Bypass Surgery?

The bypass procedure involves, first, removing sections of vein from the patient's leg that are to be used as grafts. The surgeon first attaches the vein graft to the aorta, the fountain of rapidly flowing blood, and then to the diseased arteries downstream of the blockage. The heart muscle, at least theoretically, now receives fresh blood flowing through the graft that "bypasses" the blockage, hence the name.

The original intent of this operation was to relieve the severe chest pain of angina pectoris that severely limits activity and is particularly frightening to heart patients. The operation did indeed relieve this chest pain. With this first blush of success, many physicians arbitrarily *assumed* that the operation would also prevent heart attacks and prolong life. This assumption seemed to be reasonable, but as we now know, it was, for the most part, incorrect. Despite the lack of evidence in support of this assumption, the stage was set for uncontrolled growth in this procedure—and in my opinion, for considerable abuse and a tremendous amount of unnecessary surgery. Let's now isolate the points of controversy surrounding the bypass operation.

Does the Bypass Operation Prolong Life?

One has to say at this juncture that for the majority of those receiving the operation the answer is no. In order to assess the role that any therapy has on longevity, a group of individuals with the same severity of disease must be divided evenly, with half the patients receiving the therapy, the other half not. It is important that the patients be followed at the same time. In the early days of bypass surgery many physicians claimed that the operation saved lives, for the death rate of those receiving the operation in the midseventies was lower than the death rate of similar patients in 1960 before the operation was available. This did not, however, take into account the declining death rate from heart disease in general nor the im-

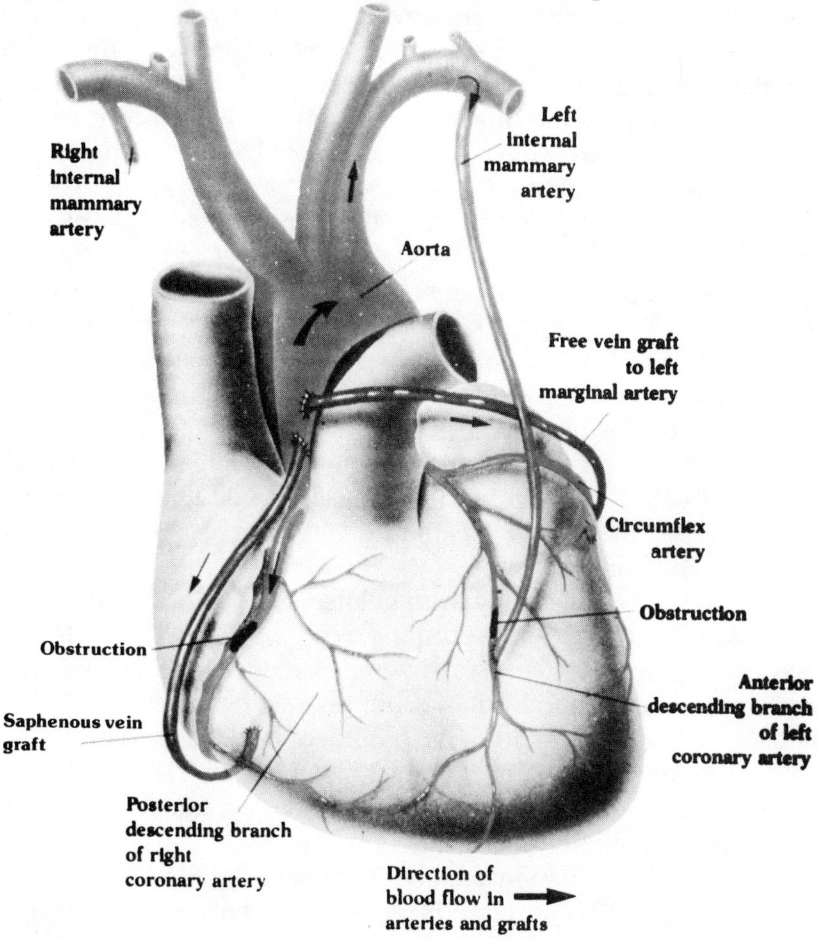

CORONARY ARTERY GRAFTS

Two vein sections from the legs and the left internal mammary artery are used above to complete a triple bypass.

provements in medical management that had occurred over that time.

In spite of the enormous number of bypass operations done, only a few controlled studies have been carried out on a very small number of patients. One of the most important was the Veterans Administration Hospital study in which thirteen separate hospitals participated. Six hundred and eighty-six patients with stable angina (angina pain that had not changed significantly over six months) were randomized, half receiving surgery and the other half treated medically. An early and clear benefit of surgery was demonstrated for patients with a blockage in the left main coronary artery. The left main coronary artery is only an inch or so long but is the trunk artery that branches into the left anterior descending artery and the left circumflex artery, which together supply blood to almost all of the heart muscle on the left side.

Because the left main artery is the source of blood for most of the muscle of the left side of the heart, blockages in this artery are indeed very dangerous. Therefore, it has been shown that blockages in the left main artery are a clear indication for bypass surgery. Fortunately, blockages in this artery are very rare, occurring in only 3 to 6 percent of the patients who undergo angiograms.

For the rest of the patients in this study, those without blockages in the left main coronary artery, there was no significant difference in those treated with surgery and those treated without surgery. After thirty-six months the death rate and heart attack rate in both groups were about the same.

The results of this study were published in 1977, at a time when the bypass operation was becoming very popular, well on its way to becoming the most common operation in medical history. It had already developed a following of both cardiologists and surgeons, who seemed so committed to its "assumed" benefits as to be almost immune to the results of the Veterans Administration Hospital study, which indicated that for many the operation just might not be life-saving or have long-term benefits.

After publication of this study, Dr. Eugene Braunwald from Harvard warned in 1977 in his editorial which appeared in *The New England Journal of Medicine:*

> An even more insidious problem is that what might be considered an industry is being built around this operation: the creation of facilities for

open heart operations in community hospitals in which no other cardiac procedures are performed, and the enlargement of surgical facilities in teaching hospitals, the proliferation of catheterization and angiographic suites as well as facilities for performing screening exercise electrocardiograms, and expansion and development of training opportunities, clinical cardiology, cardiovascular surgery, and cardiovascular radiology. This rapidly growing enterprise is developing a momentum and constituency of its own, and as time passes it will be progressively more difficult and costly to curtail it materially if the results of carefully designed studies of its efficacy prove this step to be necessary.

In spite of the study and Dr. Braunwald's call for a slowdown in the use of this procedure, rapid growth continued unchecked from 70,000 procedures done in 1977 to 170,000 done in 1982. This operation today has become the "treatment of choice" or the "accepted treatment" for a very large number of patients with various degrees of heart disease—on the yet-to-be-proved assumption that it offers the best chance to prevent a heart attack or prolong life. In fact, the procedure is so widely accepted that those physicians who advise and utilize the more conservative methods face an increased liability for malpractice in the event of a poor result.

Surely the most important study of the benefits of bypass surgery ever published was the CASS (Coronary Artery Surgery Study), funded by the National Heart, Lung, and Blood Institute at a cost of over 24 million dollars. From August 1975 until May 1979, 780 patients were carefully screened and selected from a registry of 16,626 angiogram patients from eleven different surgical centers. These patients were carefully selected to represent those with stable angina, good heart function, and with a significant blockage in one, two, or three of the major arteries supplying blood to the heart. Half of the the patients underwent surgery and the other half were treated conservatively.

The results were published in 1983 and 1984. In no group did bypass surgery demonstrate any improvement in longevity or incidence of heart attacks over the group treated only with medication. In fact, the death rate for heart patients in all three groups treated without surgery was so low that the bypass could do little to improve on it for patients of this type. The annual mortality rate of those in the medical group was only 1.6 percent, which was not significantly different from the 1.1 percent of the surgical group. Even in what is considered to be a particularly dangerous group of patients, those with triple-vessel disease, medical therapy had a mortality rate of only 2.1 percent. At death rates of only 2 percent per year without surgery, in five years 90 percent of the patient population would predictably still be alive.

For the sake of argument let's assume that bypass surgery reduced the death rate in this group of patients by 50 percent. What would that mean? That would mean that rather than having a death rate around 2 percent a year, the death rate would be around 1 percent. Is this such a dramatic difference? This would mean that in order to save one life per year, one hundred patients would have to undergo the procedure, suffer the consequences of the brain damage, endure a significant complication rate, which reaches one-third of the patients in various centers, all to save one life. But in reality, the operation is not even that successful, as the death rates were the same in both groups.

I cannot overemphasize the importance of CASS. First, it was the largest, most expensive, and most carefully designed study in which very specific questions were asked and very specific and meaningful answers were obtained. Second, controlled studies of this type cost a lot of money and require at least five years of follow-up to obtain meaningful information. This was the last such study that was in progress regarding the relative benefits of bypass surgery. As Dr. Braunwald pointed out in an editorial in the *New England Journal of Medicine:* "The importance of CASS is underscored by the fact that so far as I am aware, there are no other large, ongoing, randomized clinical trials examining this problem. If one were begun at this time [1984] it would be a decade before meaningful results would be available. Therefore, we shall have to live with the results of CASS for a long time."

In spite of the inability of bypass surgery to prolong life in the very significant group of patients that were studied in CASS, there is another group for whom the bypass operation may indeed prolong life. These are patients that do have significant blockages in their arteries as well as some damage to the heart muscle itself. It seems that the degree of damage to the heart muscle cannot be more than moderate if the bypass is to be beneficial. If heart-muscle damage is severe, the surgery does not help—and has even been shown to worsen the condition. If the heart muscle is strong, medical therapy seems as effective a treatment as the operation for most, and the surgery offers no longevity benefit. Ironically, one of the major indicators of benefit for long-term survival is not the degree of blockage in the coronary arteries but the degree of damage that has already occurred in heart muscle.

Both the Veterans Hospital study and CASS are being continued and are defining more clearly small groups of patients in whom the operation seems to prolong life. Also, these control studies are defining groups of patients in whom the surgery seems to reduce survival rate over time. For instance, in patients who have two blockages, yet have good strong heart function, the operation actually increases their death rate seven years after surgery. Had we known all of this before the operation became so popular, literally hundreds of thousands of men and women could have avoided the surgery altogether and done just as well.

In reality, what we have done with this particular form of therapy is rather bizarre. Over the last fifteen years we have subjected close to a million people to this costly and damaging operation and are now trying to figure out who it helped! The overwhelming number of patients who received this procedure consented to it believing that it was necessary either to prevent a heart attack or prolong their life. At no time, however, has there ever been *substantial* evidence that the majority of patients who received the surgery should expect long-term benefits. As late as 1978, Dr. Henry McIntosh, of Methodist Hospital and Baylor College, Houston, Texas, reviewed all of the scientific literature published on bypass surgery from 1967 through 1977. In this article published in *Circulation* (March 1978), he concluded that "available data in the literature do not indicate that the initial symptomatic improvement necessarily persists or that myocardial infarction [heart attacks], arrhythmias, or congestive heart failure will be prevented or that life will be prolonged in the vast majority of operated patients."

If one uses the criterion that the operation is needed only for those in whom it has been clearly and unequivocably shown to increase longevity *significantly,* then this surgery would be indicated only for a very small percentage, perhaps 10 to 20 percent, of those now receiving it.

Before we continue the discussion of the relative merits of the bypass operation, it is appropriate to discuss how advancements in surgery follow quite a different path than do advancements with new drugs. The development and utilization of a new drug initially requires extensive animal testing to determine whether the drug is both safe *and* effective for use in humans for a specific condition. Once these animal tests are completed, carefully controlled, human tests are also required in which the drug is slowly and painstakingly studied for *both* its effectiveness and its side effects long before it is released by the Food and Drug Administration for routine use by physicians. There are many authorities who complain that the FDA is too slow in releasing new drugs for routine use. This may or may not be so, but even with the delays and careful testing, many drugs that are released turn out to be more dangerous than suspected, inflict considerable damage, and ultimately are banned from use.

Advances in surgery have no such protocol or controls. If surgical operations are tested in animal research, it is done mostly to perfect the technique of the operation, not so much to assess its dangers or ultimate usefulness. Many, if not all, new surgical techniques are developed on the "assumption" that they might help. They are then "tried" on human beings to see if the operation works. More than thirty different surgical procedures have been employed in the past years to relieve angina and improve myocardial blood supply in patients with heart disease. All thirty of these procedures have since been abandoned, but not before thousands of patients had received them. A few of these procedures we now view with horror, as they were particularly mutilating.

Therefore, the amount of unnecessary surgery that a culture endures at any given time can only be determined as a historical fact. The trial-and-error proving ground for a surgical procedure is always the patients who receive it, and like their physicians, these patients *always* assume—even believe—that the operation is necessary, helpful, and worth the risks.

I personally believe that new surgical procedures should be subjected to the same type of controls that are now in place and widely accepted by the medical profession for new drugs. A particular surgical operation should first be done on animal models of the disease to determine both its effectiveness and safety in the animal. (We can produce almost all of our human ailments in animals, and in many cases by the same methods we produce the ailments in ourselves—poor eating habits.) If these animal experiments demonstrate a significant benefit, then carefully controlled studies in human volunteers would follow. These volunteers would all have the disease in question and would be fully informed of the potential risks and possible benefits of the operation. Half of the volunteers would receive the operation while the other half would be followed conservatively for a period of five years to determine if the procedure does indeed alter the natural course of the disease or have significant benefit. In addition, careful monitoring and follow-up of the damage that is done by the operation would be necessary. For instance, as we shall see, the heart-lung machine that is necessary for bypass surgery definitely does damage to all who are exposed to it.

If, after these studies, the operation appears to have significant benefits that are worth the damage it inflicts, then and only then would the procedure be released to the surgical community for general use in patients. Special surgical centers would be set up to provide training for the new technique to those who would then employ it.

It is my opinion that if the bypass operation had been subjected to this form of preliminary protocol prior to its general usage, the operation would never have reached the public.

Do not interpret this discussion as a blanket criticism of surgery or of surgeons. I feel that many of our surgeons are among the most caring, competent, and concerned physicians in the country. Nevertheless, their craft is so dangerous that simply allowing procedure after procedure to be developed in medical centers across the country, then abandoned to be followed by other procedures, doesn't make any sense.

You may not agree with this assessment or suggestion, nor, perhaps, will your physician. However, I suggest that you do the following: ask your physician what he would think of a pill used for the treatment of heart disease—a pill that you would take only one time; that had never been studied in either animals or humans to determine what its long-term benefits were, but which was known to be extremely dangerous, with a 2- to 10-percent death rate from the pill alone; that was a known cause of brain damage, much of it permanent, as well as a host of other problems including bleeding, infection, pulmonary embolus, and swelling and pain in the legs; and which, in addition, would cost about $25,000.00. What would he think of using this pill before any controlled studies were ever carried out! Go ahead, ask.

Let's now discuss the subjective benefits of bypass surgery.

Does the Bypass Operation Relieve Pain? If So, How?

The answer to this is yes—in 70 to 85 percent of patients pain is relieved. Yet the mechanism for that pain relief is not yet understood; there are four equally plausible theories. The first and obvious explanation is increased circulation. Blood flow now rapidly courses through the graft over the blockage, nourishing the heart that was hurting because of lack of blood. With this increased nourishment the anginal pain disappears. This is the only mechanism of pain relief that patients or doctors generally discuss, as it fits the assumptions of what the operation does.

Secondly, the operation itself causes heart attacks and these heart attacks can relieve chest pain. A heart attack that occurs during the surgery, called a perioperative infarction (*perioperative* meaning associated with surgery), is identical to the familiar heart attack that occurs so frequently in our culture. Both result in death of sections of heart muscle. If the section of heart muscle that dies during surgery was responsible for the anginal pain, no more anginal pain!

The frequency of this heart damage as a result of surgery has been measured at 40 percent in some studies. It should be noted, however, that the sensitivity of the method of measurement determines whether or not heart damage is detected. For instance, if one uses only changes in the electrocardiogram as an indication of heart-muscle damage, then the frequency of heart attacks caused by the operation will appear very low. If, on the other hand, one uses not only the changes in the electrocardiogram but also significant enzyme changes that occur with heart-muscle damage, then the frequency of damage increases substantially. It is also possible that the bypass causes a degree of heart-muscle damage that would escape any method of measurement that we currently have. Therefore, one cannot say for sure under any circumstances exactly how much or how little heart-muscle damage occurs as a result of the operation, but we know for sure that it can and does occur. In 1975, E. D. Mundth stated in the *New England Journal of Medicine* that "although some patients may be benefited in terms of relief of angina by postoperative infarction, the occurrence of an infarction has a definite adverse effect in the long-term functional results of longevity."

Thirdly, this operation could relieve chest pain by disrupting the nerve supply of the heart. The heart has a thin membranous sac covering it, called the pericardium, and in this sac are incorporated nerves that form the pain pathways from the heart. The pericardium and these nerves have to be cut during the operation to expose the heart for graft placement. Therefore, a substantial part of pain relief would likely result from this nerve resection. Relieving the pain this way is like relieving a pain in the foot by cutting certain nerves in the leg. The injury to the foot is still there, but you don't feel it.

The fourth and perhaps the most significant reason for the pain relief of the operation is the placebo effect. A placebo is a medication or therapy that has no effect upon the disease, but because the individual receiving the therapy believes strongly that the therapy is beneficial, benefits do occur. Most of these benefits are subjective benefits such as pain relief. Therefore, the measurement of a therapy on the basis of subjective improvements must take into account that the therapy could be acting as a placebo only.

We often think of the sugar pill as a placebo, but surgical procedures are the most powerful placebos ever, because of the patients' emotional involvement. In many cases, dramatic surgery is similar to the powerful faith-healing rituals of ancient medicine. In his book *The Clay Pedestal,* Dr. Thomas Preston, professor of medicine at the University of Washington and director of cardiology at the U.S. Public Health Service Hospital, Seattle, Washington, describes this surgical placebo effect:

Patients today undergo the same sort of ceremony when they have coronary bypass surgery. They spend several days at the temple (hospital) prior to the ultimate healing act. During this time they are given much encouragement; they are told of how they will be cured; they are prepared with special diets and purging; they read pamphlets . . . describing the cure; and they receive news of the cure from patients who have preceded them. On the night before the cure they are taken to the scene of the ceremony, the method of the cure is described to them, and they are shown where they will awaken afterwards. There are very few patients who are not convinced that they will be cured by the eve of their bypass operation. When it is time for the operation they are taken to the inner chamber of the temple and put to sleep. They awaken healed. The emotional response to the preparation for the operation and the intense belief that it will cure them are undoubtedly as effective as the rituals of the Aesculapian priests were. When a patient responds to the ritual, today as three thousand years ago, and is told that the specific act—the operation—caused the healing, he is deceived, for the healing power of this experience resides in the patient's mind.

More succinctly Dr. E. G. Dimond, University of Kansas Medical Center, Kansas City, Kansas, says about the placebo reaction of heart surgery:

The frightened, poorly informed man with angina, winding himself tighter and tighter, sensitizing himself to every twinge of chest discomfort, who then comes into the environment of a great medical center and a powerful, positive personality and sees and hears the results to be anticipated from the suggested therapy is not the same total patient who leaves that institution with the trademark scar.

It is my personal belief that the placebo reaction of coronary bypass surgery alone could explain the degree of pain relief achieved by this procedure. What we will never know, however, is the exact contribution of the above four mechanisms.

Regardless of how pain is relieved, an individual patient's response to this relief is often dramatic. Hardly a day goes by that I do not hear of some individual who was resurrected by bypass surgery. Prior to surgery, he was a frightened, fearful invalid unable to participate in life, and after surgery he was back on the golf course extolling the virtues of the therapy. It is hard not to be enthusiastic about a procedure that can have this effect upon an individual. It would seem that the subjective benefits alone would be reason enough for surgery if this were the rule following this operation.

The CASS, which we have already discussed, set out to determine what effect bypass surgery did have on activity level. Over a five-year period they found that the group of patients who received the surgery required less medication after surgery, but there was no significant change in either their recreational or occupational activities in comparison to the group treated without surgery. This finding was particularly surprising to many of us who awaited the results of CASS. Apparently for every patient who is "resurrected" by bypass surgery, there is another patient who received no significant subjective benefit or is even more debilitated after bypass.

Does the Pain Relief Last?

No. The one genuine effect of bypass surgery, pain relief, is fleeting. Since the surgery has no effect upon the process of atherosclerosis—in fact, actually accelerates atherosclerosis—the disease progresses and the chest pains return at a predictable rate.

In 1978, Dr. Stuart Seides, associate professor of medicine and cardiology at George Washington University and consultant to the National Institute of Health, studied records of a group of surgical patients over a period averaging five years. Three to nine months after surgery, 73 percent of this group were pain free and 27 percent had only mild symptoms. In five years, however, only 23 percent were pain free, 45 percent had mild symptoms, and 32 percent had severe symptoms which were not present at all a few months after surgery. Almost all studies on long-term results of the bypass show significant deterioration with time and generally a return of pain at rates between 5 and 15 percent per year. It is a sad patient who finds himself back in the cardiologist's office with the same pain in his chest only two or three years after the great drama of bypass surgery, but it happens quite frequently.

The Bypass Grafts Accelerate Atherosclerosis

The bypass operation does nothing to stop the process of atherosclerosis, which will continue as long as the blood is loaded with cholesterol and fat. However, those arteries that have received the grafts undergo an accelerated degree of atherosclerosis because of the blood flow brought on by the graft itself. Dr. B. J. Maurer, of the University of Alabama Medical Center in Birmingham, found that total occlusion was sixteen times more frequent in arteries that had received bypass grafts than in arteries that had been left alone. Dr. L. S. C. Griffith, Johns Hopkins Medical Center, reported that arteries with grafts developed complete blockage in 40 percent of the cases, while those without grafts went on to complete blockage in only 6 percent of those studied.

Actually we have known for years that the grafts would increase the rate of atherosclerosis in the artery that received it. However, this has not stopped the practice of many surgeons putting in more and more grafts. Their intent is to achieve "maximum revascularization" on the assumption that this would protect the patient in the years to come. It now seems, however, that this practice may have put many patients in more jeopardy, rather than less. Drs. W. Linda Cashin and David H. Blankenhorn, University of Southern California School of Medicine, studied eighty-five men who had undergone coronary bypass surgery. In this group thirty-seven arteries with minimal atherosclerosis, defined as less than 50-percent blockage, had grafts placed. After an average of thirty-seven months they found that those arteries which received the grafts had a significant progression of atherosclerosis ten times more frequently than arteries of similar blockage that did not receive the surgical graft. They then calculated that the arteries of 50-percent blockage, if not bypassed, would be more likely to deliver blood to the heart over a three-year period than would the bypass graft. Again, this demonstrates that the practice of medicine by "assumption" is always dangerous for patients who receive the therapy. Many patients who have had grafts placed in only minimally diseased vessels will possibly suffer the consequences of accelerated atherosclerosis. We cannot go back now and take out those grafts. In fact, it seems that the practice of "maximum revascularization" will even increase for some time before it begins to decrease.

What Is the Fate of the Bypass Graft Itself?

The bypass grafts are usually segments of vein that are grafted into sick arteries. Veins are much softer than arteries and in order to stay open they need a brisk flow of blood. Therefore, if the artery receiving the blood flow from the graft is diseased and there is poor flow through the graft, the graft will often close within the first few months after surgery. Even when put in place by top surgeons, 10 to 20 percent of the grafts collapse within the first year. There are literally thousands of patients who have had one, two, in some cases all of their grafts close within one year after surgery.

The tendency for these grafts to close soon after surgery is obviously a serious problem. In an attempt to reduce this early graft closure, Dr. James H. Chesebro, Mayo Clinic and Mayo Clinic Foundation in Rochester, Minnesota, studied the use of dipyridamole, a mild anticoagulant, used to keep the blood thin. In 343 patients who underwent bypass surgery, half of them received this medication before and after surgery. Eleven to eighteen months after the surgery, he found that those that received the medication had a graft-closure rate of 11 percent, while those not receiving the medication had a graft closure of 25 percent. Since patients generally receive more than one graft, Dr. Chesebro reported that there was at least one graft closed in 22 percent of the patients who received the medication while 47 percent of those who did not receive the medication had complete closure of at least one graft!

If the graft stays open for the first year, it then becomes subject to the same process of atherosclerosis that takes place in the rest of the artery. Unless the patient's physician takes steps to radically reduce the cholesterol in his patient, the graft will close at about the same rate as, if not faster than, the arteries in the heart.

Is There Risk of Death with the Bypass Operation?

Obviously there is a risk of death with any surgical procedure. The risk of death from the bypass *in the best centers* ranges between 1 and $3^1/_2$ percent. These major university centers do a tremendous volume of bypass surgery, but now most of this surgery is done in community hospitals all across the country. These hospitals will never have the volume of surgery that is achieved in the largest university centers, yet patients who receive surgery in their community hospital are generally told that their risk is the same risk reported in the largest surgical centers. This is very unlikely. It is common knowledge that the big surgical centers are the most proficient and safest. This is particularly true with a procedure like bypass surgery that utilizes the heart-lung-machine pump, which, by itself, constitutes the greatest risk to the patient. The community surgeon may be excellent and extremely well trained, but if the entire team is not up to his standards, then the patient will suffer. Be that as it may, we do not know the death rates of surgery done in these community centers, for, unlike those from the large university centers, these figures are rarely published.

There are other factors that will either increase or decrease the risk of death from the procedure. Obviously those who are older or who have diabetes, more severe heart disease, obesity, lung disease, or other problems will have higher death rates from surgery. It is ironic that those individuals with the most heart disease and therefore potentially the most to gain from the surgery have the highest death rate, while those who are healthy and have the lowest surgical death rates often have the least to gain from the operation.

Inherent Danger—the Heart-Lung Machine

As we have mentioned, in order to do the bypass, the heart is stopped for forty-five to ninety minutes while the grafts are placed, and the heart-lung machine takes over the function of both organs. Blood is detoured out of the body through the machine, where oxygen is bubbled into the blood before it goes back into the arterial system.

The heart-lung machine is a monument to the high technology of the present era, but this machine is also enormously disruptive to the human system. Blood is taken out of the body through a large vein in the lower abdomen and often is pumped back into the body through an artery also in the lower abdomen. This reverses the blood flow in the large aorta in the abdomen. Normally blood flows downward from the chest to the legs, but on the heart-lung machine it flows upward from the legs to the chest and up to the brain. Obviously, cholesterol plaques are located in the aorta and this immediate reversal in the direction of blood flow can cause cholesterol plaques to break off, and these are then carried in the blood to other organs, including the brain.

Dr. D. L. Price, Department of Neurology, Harvard Medical School, reported in 1970 the case of a bypass patient who never regained consciousness after the operation and died shortly after. An autopsy revealed that 35 percent of his brain had been destroyed by a shower of cholesterol particles. Dr. Price then reviewed thirty-five other bypass patients and found evidence of brain damage in 33 percent. The signs of brain damage reported by Dr. Price included abnormal reflexes, weakness on one side of the body, visual disturbances, and gross loss of intellectual ability. Anytime there is blockage of capillaries for any reason, you can expect problems to result.

Stirring up emboli, however, is not the only problem caused by the heart-lung machine. The blood carries specialized proteins called immunoglobulins that are part of the body's defense system. These proteins are activated by viruses, bacteria, or any foreign substance. In the activated form, they attach themselves to the foreign substance, destroying it and thus protecting the body. When blood is circulated through the heart-lung machine, these immunoglobulins become activated and are then pumped back into the body. However, these activated proteins don't know what to attack, so like mutinous soldiers, they do damage to the normal cells of the body. In 1981, Dr. D. E. Chenoweth measured the level of activated immunoglobulins in patients after bypass and found that the heart-lung machine dramatically increased their level.

Since these proteins do attack normal cells of the body it explains, at least in part, what is known as the "postpump syndrome" sometimes seen in patients after bypass surgery. The postpump syndrome results from damage that occurs to the lungs, liver, kidney, and brain after the surgery and can be fatal or leave the patient severely disabled. It is frightening to realize that the postpump syndrome is a result of the heart-lung-machine pump and has nothing to do with the skill of the surgeon or with the surgery that is taking place on the heart itself.

Brain Damage—Widely Inflicted, Generally Overlooked

Cardiologists and cardiovascular surgeons are highly skilled specialists who often focus their attention only on the heart. In many cases, they are just not aware of the myriad symptoms widely experienced by patients after bypass surgery.

It is common knowledge that many bypass patients have a period of disorientation immediately following surgery. They may have hallucinations, seizures, or other evidence of central nervous system dysfunction. When Barney Clark, the recipient of the first artificial heart, had a seizure and lapsed into a coma a week after surgery, a spokesman for the hospital said that this was not unusual in patients having undergone heart surgery. Indeed, it is quite common and is brought on primarily by the heart-lung-machine pump.

In most cases, the obvious brain dysfunctions are temporary, but permanent damage is to some degree inflicted and often goes unnoticed. Assessment of the degree of brain damage depends upon the sensitivity of the measurement. For instance, many heart surgeons not fully aware of the degree of brain damage that results from the heart-lung machine would likely state that brain damage following bypass surgery was rare. The sensitivity of this method of assessing the degree of brain damage is very low, but if sensitive tests are done on patients both before and after surgery, a different picture arises.

Dr. Torkel Åberg, Department of Thoracic Surgery, University Hospital, Uppsala, Sweden, did elaborate psychometric tests on 113 open-heart-surgery patients one week before, one week after, and two months after their operations. These sensitive tests measured various intellectual functions. Fourteen of these patients (12 percent) had obvious brain damage, such as a stroke which led to gross brain dysfunction and alteration in the intellectual test. However, the remaining 99, who had no obvious brain damage, also showed marked disturbances on the intellectual test given two months after surgery. There were significant changes in the visual, spatial ability; in perceptual speed; and in visual/spatial cognition (cognition is a process of knowing something). There was less significant loss of logical perception in memory. These changes did not occur in another group of 45 percent who had undergone major chest surgery but without the use of the heart-lung machine.

Two recent studies have indicated that brain damage occurs to some extent in everyone that undergoes this operation. Dr. Leif Henriksen, Department of Neurology and Thoracic Surgery, State University Hospital in Copenhagen, Denmark, measured blood flow in the brain in thirty-seven patients before and after bypass surgery. He found in every case a reduction in blood flow after the surgery, indicating at least some postoperative brain damage. He made identical measurements of brain blood-flow in patients who underwent chest surgery but were not put on the heart-lung-machine pump, and he found no changes either before or after surgery. He concluded that the blood flow "changes that occurred after extracorporeal [heart-lung-machine pump] circulation in our patients were clearly pathological and did not occur postoperatively in the control. Extracorporeal circulation affects the gray matter evenly." The gray matter in the brain houses intellectual function and certain aspects of personality. The fact that the reduced blood flow represents damage throughout this section of the brain is particularly frightening.

In a more recent study by Dr. Torkel Åberg it was found that in thirty-three out of thirty-six patients undergoing open heart surgery and subjected to the heart-lung-machine pump, the enzyme adenylate kinase was elevated in the cerebrospinal fluid that covers the brain. Elevation of this enzyme indicates brain damage. He also found that the enzyme level correlated with the degree of intellectual dysfunction demonstrated after surgery.

Therefore, depending upon the sensitivity of the measurement, the heart-lung machine begins to inflict damage to the brain and to all the other organs the minute it is turned on. The longer one stays hooked up to the heart-lung machine the more severe is the damage. Secondly, the elderly and more severely ill patients are more susceptible to the damage brought on by the heart-lung machine. One should never underestimate the danger of this operation, but rarely is the potential for brain damage ever openly discussed with the patients. As I mentioned, many heart specialists focus so intently on the functions of the heart that they miss the complications of this operation endured by their patients.

One example of this was the case of one of my patients who enrolled in our Institute several years after having had bypass surgery. The police chief in a small Southern California town, he was subjected to a double bypass because of rather dubious chest pains. After surgery he had such memory loss that his functioning on the job changed dramatically. For instance, he would give conflicting orders: after giving instructions to one individual, he would then order someone else to do something entirely different about the situation or cancel the order completely. This obviously disrupted the function of the police station, and it was his secretary who finally told him of the conflicting orders he was giving and the change in his personality since the surgery.

Before surgery he had been a much-sought-after public speaker, speaking to groups of 50 to 5,000. After surgery he gave up public speaking entirely because of word loss, faulty speech, and feelings of insecurity. After surgery he developed sleep disorders, sleeping no more than two hours without waking up. There was also a marked change in his temperament: before the operation he had been mild mannered and even tempered, but after the operation he was prone to outbursts of temper of such severity that he had to warn individuals around him not to take them personally. After surgery there was a marked decrease in his ability to add and subtract rapidly and a reduction in other forms of abstract thinking and functioning. In short, the damage inflicted upon his brain by the heart-lung machine had dramatically altered his professional, social, and intellectual functioning. Yet his cardiologist and his cardiovascular surgeon were totally unaware of these changes. When I questioned him about these changes in his personality and intellectual function, he told me that he thought they were due to premature senility.

Why Is the Bypass Operation So Popular?

In view of all the negative reports on the bypass operation, the trauma that it inflicts on every patient who receives it, and the studies that clearly show that it fails to produce long-term benefits for the majority of those who receive it, you might ask yourself at this juncture: Why is the operation so popular? There are three possible answers to this question.

One obvious answer would be that this procedure generates a lot of money. Every step leading to the bypass operation is profitable for those providing the services. The profit motive is at work in almost every endeavor in this country. This in itself is not bad but we are reticent to recognize the profit motive as a force when it comes to the practice of medicine. Doctors are supposed to be above the profit motive in making their decisions, and surely, most physicians are. There are also physicians who are excessively motivated by profit. As in every profession, there is a variety of individuals with extremes of motivation. It is not my intention to discuss this sensitive subject at any great length, but I would pose two questions to you the reader. First, the data to date indicates that many patients who receive bypass surgery do not experience substantial long-term benefit, yet this procedure nurtures in handsome manner those that are most active in using it. Do you think that the frequency of this procedure would be the same if it were not profitable to those doing it? Secondly, does it not seem odd to you that literally billions of dollars are being spent every year on a procedure that has been shown not to play any significant role in reducing the death rate of the disease that it is designed to treat?

The second reason for its popularity is that it appeals to both patient and physician, who desire to do something immediate and dramatic about the problem. This procedure looks great on paper. When the patient reviews his own angiogram and sees the location of the blockages, it is hard for him not to believe that well-placed grafts would not solve the problem. As Dr. Robert Buccino, of the Watson Clinic, Lakeland, Florida, points out:

> Most cardiologists favor an activist course of treatment. Consultants are brought in at an early stage often before simple measures are applied. Cardiologists have a tendency to encourage excessive performance of special tests and procedures thus justifying their involvement in the case of satisfying expectations of the patient, family, and referring physician. There is a bias to interpret borderline data at each point of evaluation by erring on the side of the safety—by doing more rather than less. The path of least resistance leads ultimately to the operation suite.
>
> The problem with premature or unnecessary aortocoronary bypass surgery is its potential for causing more harm than good. The indiscriminate promotion of bypass surgery is inappropriate and should be resisted except in circumstances where its use is supported by firm medical data.

A third reason for its popularity is that yesterday's assumptions have become today's beliefs. The claims of the early proponents, even though now disproven for the most part, are nevertheless believed by a large number of practicing physicians trained in the use of bypass surgery. Unlike many other heart operations that had a brief flurry of application by a limited number of physicians, the bypass procedure today is done nationwide in almost every community. Over the last fifteen years medical centers in the country have trained cardiologists and surgeons to deliver these services. For the large number of physicians who have spent several years and thousands of hours training to use this form of therapy, it is inconceivable that they should now sharply curtail its use. Also, when any form of therapy becomes widely practiced, that in itself convinces many practitioners of its usefulness. When a therapy becomes commonplace, it no longer requires proof of its usefulness. Therefore, by common consent, not proof of benefit, bypass surgery is firmly entrenched in American medicine.

If Not the Bypass, What Are the Alternatives?

Today's potential bypass recipient should realize that medical management without surgery is extremely successful for most and consistent with a low death rate. Drs. Philip Podrid, Thomas Graboys, and Bernard Lown from Harvard Medical School reported their experience with 212 patients whose stress tests indicated they had severe heart disease. The overwhelming majority of cardiologists in the country would have referred almost all of these men for an angiogram, which would have led most into the operating room. This Harvard group, however, treated them with appropriate medications, mild exercise, and mild dietary changes. The yearly death rate was only 1.4 percent—which is lower than the death rate from surgery alone. These researchers concluded: "There is rarely a need to resort to cardiac surgery; medical management is highly successful and associated with a low mortality."

Summary: Who Should Have the Bypass

There is no question those patients that have a clearly defined and significant blockage in the left main coronary artery, the short artery that supplies blood to the left side of the heart, should have the operation.

It seems that patients who have severe chest pain that is unresponsive to medical therapy and who seek surgery for relief of this pain are also true candidates.

Other patients may benefit from this surgery, including those who have mildly reduced heart function and significant blockages in three major arteries, and those with a combination of two indicators of risk—resting electrocardiogram changes, history of heart attack, or history of high blood pressure.

In looking at these subgroups of patients one cannot say for sure that the surgery is always the best way to go. It took seven years to define this group, and during that time improvements in the method of conservative management have also taken place, not the least of which is the recognition that vigorous dietary changes are much more powerful a treatment for heart disease than was ever thought.

Except for those with left main-artery disease, any decision to have this operation should take into account the risk and the actual damage that occurs in everyone who is subjected to this surgery. Patients should be made aware of the reality of the brain damage and other well-documented complications that are a part of this method of handling the disease. Once permanent damage is done, neither the doctor nor the patient can retrace their steps and make another decision. If patients, when given the full disclosure of the risk inherent in this procedure, do not wish to undergo surgery, then physicians should definitely support them in their decision and help to orchestrate a program not only of appropriate medication but also of vigorous dietary cholesterol control. I believe that patients in the high-risk groups should not be threatened with abandonment if they indeed wish to defer surgery and are well informed. It is for these patients that this book has such value, for the dietary regime included will surely help to lower the blood cholesterol level.

Included at the end of this chapter are several important references that I believe every potential bypass patient should read and discuss with his/her cardiologist. These references can be obtained with your physician's help at any medical library. It would take less than two hours for you to read them in their entirety and certainly less time to read only their summaries and conclusions. Secondly, it should take about one hour for you to discuss with your physician the content of these references and how your particular condition fits with those described in the literature. The decision to have bypass surgery is possibly one of the most important decisions of your life and should not be made without your clear understanding of the risk and benefits of this particular approach.

References

Åberg, Torkel, M.D., et al. Release of adenylate kinase into the cerebral spinal fluid during open heart surgery and its relation to post-operative intellectual function. *The Lancet.* 1139–1142, May 22, 1982.

Braunwald, Eugene, M.D. Coronary artery surgery at the crossroads. An editorial. *New England Journal of Medicine.* 297: 661–663, 1977.

Braunwald, Eugene, M.D. Editorial retrospective, effects of coronary artery bypass grafting on survival; implications of the randomized coronary artery surgery study. *New England Journal of Medicine.* 309: 1181–1184, 1983.

Cashin, W. Linda, M.D., et al. Accelerated progression of atherosclerosis in coronary vessels with minimal lesions that are bypassed. *New England Journal of Medicine.* 311: 824–828, 1984.

Coronary artery surgery study (CASS). Myocardial infarction and mortality in the CASS randomized trial. *New England Journal of Medicine.* 310: 750–758, 1984.

Coronary artery surgery study (CASS). A randomized trial of coronary artery bypass surgery, quality of life in patients randomly assigned to treatment groups. *Circulation.* 68: 951–960, 1983.

Coronary artery surgery study (CASS). A randomized trial of coronary artery bypass surgery, survival data. *Circulation.* 68: 939–950, 1983.

Henriksen, Leif, M.D. Evidence suggestive of diffuse brain damage following cardiac operations. *The Lancet.* 816–821, April 14, 1984.

McIntosh, Henry D., M.D., and Jorge A. Garcia, M.D. The first decade of aortocoronary bypass grafting, 1967–1977. Special article, a review. *Circulation.* 57: 405–431, 1978.

Murphy, Marvin L., M.D., et al. Treatment of chronic stable angina; a preliminary report of survival data of the randomized Veterans Administration Cooperative study. *New England Journal of Medicine.* 297: 621–627, 1977.

Ornish, Dean, M.D., et al. Effects of stress management training and dietary changes in treating ischemic heart disease. *Journal of the American Medical Association.* 249: 54–59, 1983.

Podrid, Philip J., M.D., et al. Prognosis of medically treated patients with coronary artery disease with profound ST segment depression during exercise testing. *New England Journal of Medicine.* 305: 1111–1116, 1981.

Taylor, K. M., M.D. Brain damage during open heart surgery. An editorial. *Thorax.* 37: 873–876, 1982.

The Veterans Administration Coronary Artery Bypass Surgery Cooperative Study Group. Eleven-year survival in the Veterans Administration randomized trial of coronary bypass surgery for stable angina. *New England Journal of Medicine.* 311: 1333–1339, 1984.

4

Heart Disease Is Reversible

Atherosclerosis, the process that brings on heart disease, is reversible, and we know how to achieve this. Not only is atherosclerosis avoidable and preventable, but it can be turned around. Arteries obstructed with plaque can be cleared, thereby letting the blood flow again. Now this is news! Infinitely more important than some new or more elaborate techniques of managing the end stages of the disease.

The methods for reversing atherosclerosis are well established and the evidence supporting them have been gathered over the last nine decades by many doctors and scientists. The sane treatment of this ailment will become the standard treatment in time, as more and more doctors realize the power of the conservative approach, which includes vigorous diet changes like those in this book.

For some reason, the concept of reversing atherosclerosis generates heated controversy. Ironically, however, the data indicating that reversal of atherosclerosis does occur is actually stronger than the data used to support some of the more common heart disease therapies.

We have learned what we need to know about the progress and reversal of atherosclerosis from wartime observations, from animal experiments, human case studies, planned human experiments, and observations with the use of oxygen.

Wartime Observations

War is hell, but sometimes entire populations benefit from it in ways they never hear about. During the years of World War I and World War II the Europeans had drastic food shortages, the most noticeable being meat, eggs, milk, butter, cheese, and lard. Raising, slaughtering, processing, storing, transporting, and distributing these foods is a complex industry easily disrupted by war, and people fell back on more easily raised and stored food like potatoes, vegetables, and particularly grains which can be stored for a long time.

All through the hard years of war there were scientists observing the effects of privation which seemed to have been a blessing in disguise. During, and just after World War I, Dr. T. Ashoff reported a significant reduction of cholesterol deposits in the arteries of the civilian population which he attributed to the reduced consumption

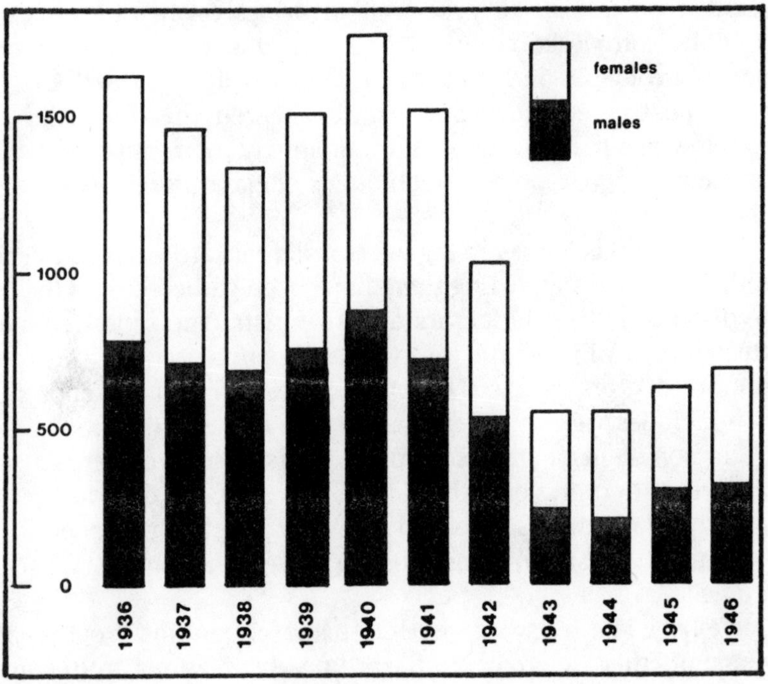

Death rate in men and women in civilian population before and during World War II. (Vartiainen, I. *Annals of Internal Medicine,* Finland, 36 (1947):748.)

of high-fat foods. More conclusive evidence was gathered in World War II. In Finland, Dr. Ilmari Vartiainen and Dr. Karl Kanerva documented a 67 percent drop in deaths due to heart disease in the civilian population as compared with pre-war days, and there was much less cholesterol plaque. The Norwegian government published similar findings during the war and the austere period following it. Routine autopsies on the civilian population showed marked reduction of cholesterol deposits. All of these researchers concluded that the decline in heart disease death was associated with reduced consumption of eggs, butter, and other foods rich in fat and cholesterol.

Dr. William Castelli, one of the chief investigators of the Framingham heart studies that showed the blood cholesterol level to be a major risk factor, took his medical degree in Belgium in the early 1950s. He had a crusty pathology professor, Eugene Picard,

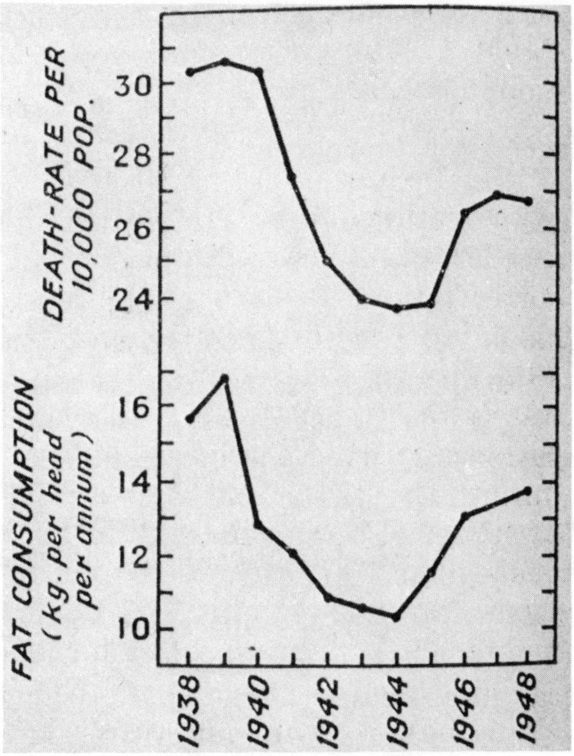

Mortality from circulatory diseases, and consumption of fat in form of butter, milk, cheese, and eggs. (Ström, Alex. "Mortality from circulatory diseases in Norway 1940–1945." *The Lancet,* January 20, 1951:128.)

who amused students by walking around mumbling "They're coming back." Someone asked him who "they" were, and Picard said "cholesterol deposits in the arteries" which were again showing up in cadavers as Belgians returned to their rich peacetime eating habits.

All this splendid wartime documentation is ignored today by defenders of the meat and dairy industries when they say that we have had no definitive, controlled, large-scale study proving that a shift to a vegetable diet will dramatically reduce atherosclerosis in human beings. If you ever hear anyone take that line, ask this: When and how could scientists ever persuade 50 million people to shift to a low-fat diet for four years? What kind of test would rival the wartime experience of Europe for conclusive results?

Animal Experiments

You have probably learned that experiments on animals are not conclusive for human beings. That is true, but again and again animal experiments do point the way for research that is beneficial for humans.

The research on atherosclerosis in animals would fill a library in itself and points clearly to high-fat and high-cholesterol foods as the major culprit. In fact, the strong relationship of dietary fat and cholesterol became apparent almost eighty years ago.

Around 1900 in Europe scientists were trying to find the causes of atherosclerosis. Something was damaging the arteries: What? In labs they injected irritating substances into rabbits. In time they killed the rabbits and sliced open their arteries. Clean. No trace of atherosclerosis in these vegetarian creatures. Rabbits on their natural diet eat almost no cholesterol and their blood cholesterol level is low—about 120 mg percent. At that level atherosclerosis does not occur.

The atherosclerosis-causing substances were discovered by accident. In 1909 the Russian scientist Ignatowski was studying the effects of high-protein foods, such as meat, milk, and eggs, on rabbit kidneys (a caged rabbit will eat meat). In due time the rabbits were dissected and, while kidney damage was nil, severe atherosclerosis was found in the arteries.

A debate ensued. Some researchers said protein caused the

artery damage, while others blamed fat and cholesterol. Anitschkow, another Russian, settled the dispute in 1913 by producing severe atherosclerosis in rabbits with a diet of fat and cholesterol, and no protein. Since that time the routine way to produce atherosclerosis in lab animals is to feed them saturated fat and cholesterol; it never fails. And no other method has ever produced the condition in animals. As Dr. William Connor of the University of Oregon has said, "If ever a human disease can be produced in animals, it is atherosclerosis, and if ever the requirements of that disease have been isolated it is fat and cholesterol in the diet."

The excitement begins when these animals are put back on their natural low-fat diet and atherosclerosis begins to reverse itself. Dr. Draga Vesselinovitch, of the University of Chicago, reported a 50 percent reduction of artery damage in monkeys after eighteen months on a low-fat diet. Not only did the cholesterol deposits dissolve but the linings of arteries were regenerating.

Reversal of atherosclerosis happens more rapidly when cholesterol-lowering agents are added to the low-fat diet. Cholestyramine and cholestipol, two such agents, are fiber-like substances called anion exchange resins that speed up the reversal. They are not absorbed into the body when ingested but pass through the intestines and out with the stool. In the intestine they attach to cholesterol molecules and carry them away, thus the lowering blood cholesterol. Certain natural fibers have the same cholesterol-eliminating effect: pectins in fruit, cellulose in vegetables, and bran in grains.

Human Case Studies

Human beings are very different from rabbits and we can't always apply to our own systems what we learn from rabbit experiments. Monkeys, on the other hand, are close to us in body structure and function and experimental results with them must be taken very seriously. Nevertheless, although reversal of atherosclerosis was easily demonstrable in monkeys, many physicians have insisted that similar reversal would not occur in human beings. They have reasoned that since blockages in humans were of long standing, they would be excessively hard due to calcium and therefore fixed and irreversible. This is reasonable, since we do know that age plays a part in the reversibility of blockages and is a point of discussion. Nonetheless, the tenacity with which some physicians—even heart specialists—have resisted the concept of any reversibility of atherosclerosis is ironic.

Dr. William Castelli, director of the Framingham heart studies, commented on this resistance in a lecture given at Loma Linda University. At numerous medical centers he has presented "before and after" angiograms of heart arteries showing that the cholesterol deposits present at one point in time had disappeared with conservative treatment aimed at achieving very low cholesterol levels. He was always amused that many cardiologists and heart surgeons would form a line at the microphone to state that the original angiogram was not a cholesterol plaque, but an involuntary spasm of the artery that only looked like a blockage. Dr. Castelli then quipped that if that were the case, a lot of patients are receiving bypass surgery for spasms of the arteries, not actual blockages!

In the fall of 1984, a prominent cardiovascular surgeon who was presenting a television show in Los Angeles discussing the bypass operation stated that reversibility of atherosclerotic blockages in the coronary arteries had never been demonstrated by angiogram. I appeared the next day on the same program with several examples of blockages in the coronary arteries that had been reversed, as demonstrated by angiogram, and these examples had been published in medical literature easily available to all physicians.

What is needed is an open and enthusiastic discussion of the various factors that we now know play a part in the reversibility of atherosclerosis. Which blockages reverse the fastest; how long does it take? What effect does age have on the process? How low must the cholesterol level be? What are the safest and most effective methods of lowering the cholesterol level? What is the role of exercise? What is the role of other drugs? In short, there should be a rich and productive dialogue. History will show, however, that those most vocally opposed to discussion of reversibility have, for the most part, been heart specialists, who should be in the forefront directing the dialogue to its most productive avenues.

In 1976, Dr. L. L. Basta reported the case of a young woman who had severe high blood pressure as a result of a 90 percent atherosclerotic blockage of the artery to her right kidney. This caused the kidney to produce hormones that raised her blood pressure.

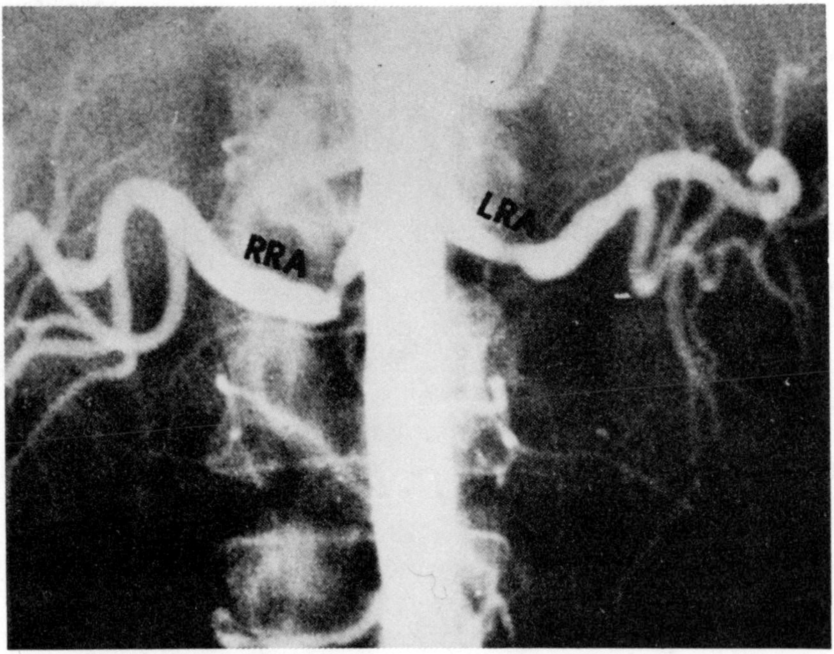

Regression of atheroslcerotic stenosing lesions of the renal arteries and spontaneous cure of systemic hypertension through control of hyperlipidemia. (Basta, L.L. *The American Journal of Medicine,* 61 (1976):421.)

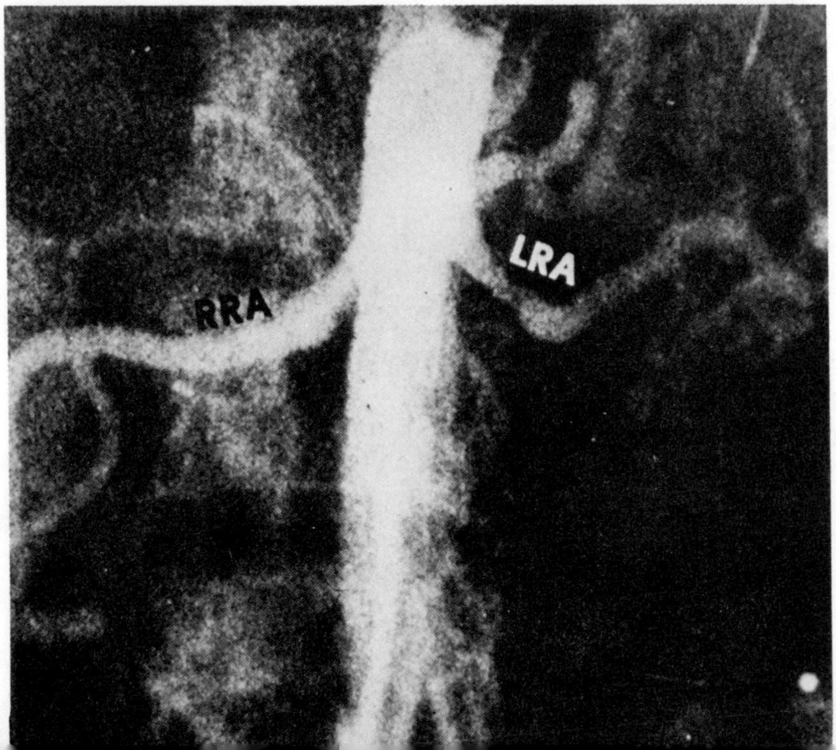

When the initial x-rays were taken that showed the blockage, blood tests showed her cholesterol level to be high—334 mg percent. A low-cholesterol diet and cholesterol-lowering medications brought her cholesterol level down to 150 to 165 mg percent. A repeat x-ray after three years on that treatment showed the artery blockage to have reversed almost completely.

Another case is reported by Dr. Thomas Bassler in 1980. A sixty-one-year-old man who had endured angina pectoris for thirteen years had an angiogram that showed one main artery blocked 95 percent, another 75 percent. An ideal bypass candidate, the man decided to cure himself by increasing his daily walking from two miles to six, and started to do some slow jogging. His angina went away in about two months. He kept up his program and at the age of sixty-eight another angiogram showed that the 95 percent blockage had shrunk to 50 percent, the 75 percent blockage to 30 percent.

In 1981 Dr. D. Roth, of the University Hospital of London, Ontario, reported the case of a forty-six-year-old attorney who was admitted to the hospital with severe chest pain and an eight-month history of angina brought on by exertion. An exercise test and a thallium scan both showed inadequate blood flow to parts of the heart and an angiogram showed a large blockage in a major artery. An excellent candidate for bypass surgery or the balloon angioplasty, he instead went home, cut down his meat and dairy intake, and increased his exercise. Six months later his chest pain was completely gone, his cholesterol level had dropped from 269 to 209, and his triglycerides (a measure of neutral fat) went from 205 to 93. A year later his heart was functioning normally and a repeat angiogram showed that the blockage had unquestionably been reversed.

Planned Human Experiments

These individual cases prove without a doubt that reversal can and does take place in human beings. However, more significant evidence comes from studies of groups of patients. In 1966 in Sweden, Dr. C. R. Öst treated thirty-one patients with blockages in the arteries to the legs using large doses of a drug called niacin (which

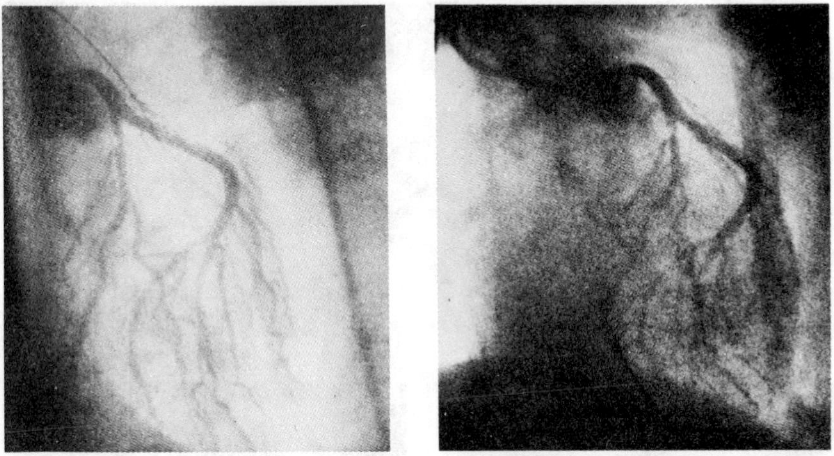

"Non-invasive and invasive demonstration of spontaneous regression of coronary artery disease." (Roth, D. *Circulation,* 62 (1980):888–896.)

I will describe later) for a period of three and a half years. Before and after angiograms showed that with the niacin treatment 10 percent of the patients had reversal, 35 percent remained stable (there was no worsening, and the process of atherosclerosis stopped), and 55 percent had progression of atherosclerosis. This study was interesting in that only one treatment method, niacin, was reported. We do not know if appropriate diet changes were recommended, but because niacin lowers the blood cholesterol level, reversal or stabilization occurred in 45 percent.

In another study by Dr. Robert Barndt and Dr. David Blankenhorn of the University of Southern California, a group of twenty-five patients with severe blockages to the legs were put on a low-fat diet and cholesterol-lowering medication. A repeat angiogram demonstrated reversal in 36 percent of the patients in only fourteen months, while 10 percent remained stable and 54 percent worsened. They were able to estimate not only how much reversal had taken place, but also the rate, or speed, of reversal.

All of these studies show that nonsurgical therapy for lowering blood levels in fat and cholesterol is the direction to follow. They also indicate that more is needed in the treatment of atherosclerosis, or perhaps a combination of things. Could one of those things be oxygen therapy?

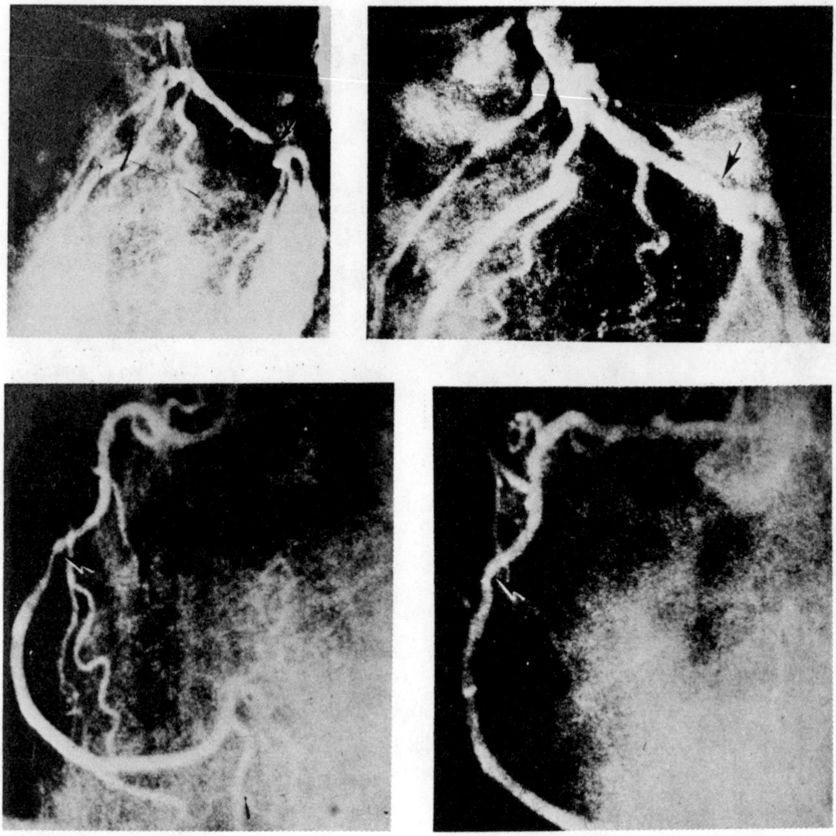

(Bassler, T. "Regression of Athroma," *Western Journal of Medicine,* 132 (1980):474–475.)

Observations with Oxygen Use

We use oxygen therapy at the Institute as part of the treatment for heart disease. Patients breathe bottled oxygen using a mask for short periods each day. Let me warn against the idea that this by itself is a fast or easy fix for atherosclerosis. That said, let's consider the role of oxygen in treating heart disease.

The air we breathe at sea level is about 21 percent oxygen, 72 percent nitrogen, and 6 to 8 percent other gases, including carbon dioxide. This percentage of oxygen is more than adequate for good health, but studies have shown that increasing oxygen intake is not only helpful in a crisis but can help to reverse atherosclerosis.

Low oxygen tension can begin and accelerate the atherosclerotic process. Chapter 7 will describe how this happens in detail. For the present, let us accept that a lower amount of oxygen in the blood than is normal is harmful, and that restoring oxygen is helpful. A high-fat diet lowers oxygen by clogging circulation. Smoking puts carbon monoxide into the blood thereby displacing oxygen in the red blood cells. Lack of exercise deteriorates the oxygen-utilizing system of the body. All this being true, the question is: Will raising the oxygen level slow the process of atherosclerosis, and perhaps help reverse it?

Dr. K. Kjeldsen, of the University of Copenhagen, Denmark, studied twenty-four rabbits that were being fed an atherosclerosis-producing diet. Twelve of the rabbits spent ten weeks in an oxygen chamber breathing air in which the normal 21 percent oxygen component was increased to 28 percent. The other twelve breathed room air for the same period. At the end of the test period the oxygen-chamber rabbits showed blood cholesterol reduced 7 percent, triglycerides 26 percent lower, the amount of cholesterol deposited in the artery 50 percent lower, and the size, shape, and degree of damage brought on by the high-fat diet was less than in animals in room air.

Furthermore, increasing the oxygen speeds up the reversal of atherosclerosis. Dr. Robert Wissler, Professor of Pathology at the University of Chicago, and one of the world's foremost experts on atherosclerosis, put a group of rabbits on a high-fat, high-cholesterol diet, producing in them high cholesterol levels and severe artery damage. The rabbits were then returned to a low-fat, low-cholesterol diet and given various other therapeutic regimens. For one group the additional treatment consisted of two hours a day of breathing 100 percent oxygen. This group showed accelerated reversal of atherosclerosis. According to Dr. Wissler, increasing the oxygen available to these rabbits accelerated the reversal of atherosclerosis by increasing the amount of oxygen available to muscle cells of the arteries. As I discuss in Chapter 7, the muscle cells of the inner one-third of our larger arteries depend on oxygen that is being carried in the blood of the artery itself. This oxygen must diffuse across the cell barrier that covers these muscle cells. When the blood oxygen levels are reduced by a high-fat diet or smoking, then these muscle cells are damaged and the process of atherosclerosis is started. Now, with a layer of cholesterol covering the artery, the muscle cells of the artery are even less likely to get adequate oxygen. By increasing the oxygen in the blood, you increase the amount of oxygen available to these cells, which would reduce their tendency to attract fat and cholesterol deposits, and even accelerate the reversal process.

Dr. R. Wissler concluded that "hyperoxia [breathing additional oxygen] is beneficial in arresting and/or reversing atherosclerosis in rabbits. Moreover, a combination of hyperoxia, low-fat diet, combined with cholestyramine . . . prove to be more effective than any of these treatments used alone. The combined treatment of this disease seems logical in view of this multifaceted pathogenesis."

I have been using supplemental oxygen as a treatment modality for atherosclerosis for close to six years, and it never ceases to "raise the eyebrows" of my fellow physicians. We all know that supplemental oxygen is a routine first step in the emergency room for any patient with chest pain, and is routinely used in the coronary care unit with patients recovering from a heart attack. To use supplemental oxygen regularly at home, however, generates a considerable amount of resistance by many who are simply unfamiliar with the fact that oxygen can be used and may be helpful for the ongoing treatment of atherosclerosis.

So What's the Answer?

From the wealth of literature on atherosclerosis there is a clearly indicated six-point program of treatment for heart disease of almost any degree of severity.

1. *Reduce the cholesterol level in the blood* to that of human beings or monkeys on a low-fat, low-cholesterol diet. That level is 150 mg percent—much lower than certain authorities will offer as a "normal" level. But it is a reachable level, with the right diet and with cholesterol-reducing substances.

2. *Stop smoking.* Carbon monoxide in the blood cancels many of the benefits of cholesterol control and lowering blood pressure. This is a very, very tough step for cigarette addicts, but is an absolute must.

3. *Control blood pressure.* High blood pressure causes damage to the arteries; when it is brought under control the arteries have a chance to repair themselves. Later I will describe how diet works to control blood pressure which is all that is necessary in most percent of high-blood-pressure cases.

4. *Exercise.* An exercise program designed for the patient's capacity and needs will protect him against atherosclerosis and can aid in reversal—but not by itself. Consider the case of Arthur Ashe, the tennis champ at Wimbledon. However, at the top of his professional career he had a heart attack and subsequently had two bypass operations in four years. Diet and cholesterol control are more important than exercise alone. Exercise can never make it safe for anyone who has high blood pressure.

5. *Supplemental oxygen.* There is no need for this if you are young or healthy, but if you are working to overcome atherosclerosis, oxygen may help. Patients at the Institute breathe oxygen for half an hour twice a day. You can read, watch TV, settle down for the night, or even ride your stationary bicycle while doing your oxygen stints. If the oxygen is humidified there is no danger except perhaps for patients with severe lung disease, but no one should use oxygen except under a doctor's care.

Home use of oxygen should only be done under your doctor's care and with his prescription. Often insurance companies and other third-party payers refuse to pay for oxygen use as a treatment for atherosclerosis. It generally doesn't fit the guidelines for oxygen use. I believe that these kind of restrictions are necessary. We should not expect a blank check from an insurance company or Medicare or any other third-party payer, but when the rationale for the use of a therapy can be validated by scientific data, then we should expect insurance companies and other third-party payers to have flexible guidelines.

If you or your physician wish to use oxygen at home as a part of your treatment protocol, we have prepared a succinct letter about its use with references that could be submitted to your insurance carriers in support of your claim. Simply write to us and request the letter on oxygen therapy reimbursement.

6. *Vitamins and minerals.* See Chapter 13. That chapter will probably stir up more comment and controversy than any other in this book. All I want to say here is (1) don't ascribe super healing qualities to vitamins and minerals and (2) don't take large doses of single vitamins because they can throw your metabolic system out of balance. But nutritional supplements make as much sense as any other aspect of altering your eating habits if they are used sensibly.

This six-point program for overcoming heart disease is sound, can be used by anyone, and should be added to your current treatment. It offers hope to people who know the pain and anxiety of heart disease and who fear the surgery route. But remember, for heart disease, there is no "quick fix."

5

Our Crazy Diet

You are what you eat
Of this have no doubt
What goes into your body
Is how you'll turn out

The American Way—Fat of the Land

Americans and Western Europeans consume a lot of fat and animal protein. The caloric composition of the American diet is very high in fat, 43 percent, 12 percent protein, and about 45 percent carbohydrate calories. The emphasis is on animal protein: eggs and bacon for breakfast, hamburger or some other protein sandwiches for lunch, and the ever present steak, fish, or chicken for dinner. We eat so much meat you'd think we were a nation of carnivorous dogs and cats, instead of humans.

What most people don't realize is that foods of animal origin are mostly caloric fat. Lean beef, for instance, is almost 40 to 60 percent caloric fat while sirloin steak is almost 85 percent fat calories. Hard cheeses referred to as a high-protein food are 65 to 85 percent fat calories while mayonnaise, most salad dressings, margarines, and butter are almost 100 percent fat calories. Second, these foods have no carbohydrates or fiber present which are both essential for optimum human health. High-fat foods are disastrous to the human system which was designed for light, low-fat vegetable foods (fruits, vegetables, legumes, seeds, and grains) that are high in carbohydrates and fiber.

Comparative Physiology: Meat Eaters versus Vegetable Eaters

In general, mammals can be separated into three different classes based upon their natural diet: meat eaters (carnivores such as lions, tigers, dogs, and cats), leaf and grass eaters (herbivores which include grazers such as horses and cows, antelopes and other large herding mammals), and fruit and vegetable eaters (monkeys, apes, and chimpanzees). When man's physical characteristics are compared to these three classes, he is obviously a fruit and vegetable eater.

Teeth and Mouth

The major difference in these three groups is found in the digestive tract which begins with the teeth and the function of the mouth. A meat eater has sharp, pointed, canine fangs ideal for piercing hide and tearing chunks of flesh from a carcass. The mouth is a major tool for both hunting and defense. For instance, the muzzled German shepherd is harmless, but without the muzzle he is formidable. The meat eater has no molars or grinding teeth and does not chew his food, but rather swallows chunks of meat whole. The meat eater also has no significant digestive enzymes in his saliva as these enzymes are generally for the breakdown of carbohydrate foods.

The teeth and mouth structure of man, however, is identical to the fruit and vegetable eaters. He does not have sharp fangs, nor is his mouth designed for hunting and defense. Man's first recourse in defense or aggression is to use his hands, not his mouth. Again, like the fruit and vegetable eater, man has well-developed molars in the back of his mouth which are needed to grind vegetables and fruit and mix them with the enzymes present in his saliva. These enzymes, ptyalin and others, are necessary to start the digestion of carbohydrates found in fruits and vegetables.

Without weapons or tools, man is neither physically nor instinctively capable of eating large amounts of meat. If meat were natural to the diet of human beings we would stalk animals in the field, catch them with our hands, bite them to death, and feast on their warm bleeding carcasses. However, human beings are not naturally bloodthirsty and our natural ability with our hands and arms as well as our instincts lead us to take an orange, strawberries, or an ear of corn and eat them with relish when hungry. In fact, most people would be sickened if they had to kill their meat themselves. We generally have someone else do the killing, and we boil, bake, or fry the meat and disguise it with all kinds of sauces and spices so that it bears no resemblance to the flesh of the animal.

I believe that one way to sharply curtail meat consumption would be to have everyone visit a slaughterhouse or meat processing plant a couple times a year. For many, one visit would be enough.

Hydrochloric Acid

The stomach of meat eaters produces twenty times the hydrochloric acid of the human stomach. This large amount of acid is necessary for the rapid digestion of animal flesh. Fruit and vegetables require much less hydrochloric acid for digestion and the human stomach complies. If we produced the same amount of hydrochloric acid as meat eaters do, we wouldn't have a stomach for very long.

The Intestinal Tract

Meat spoils (putrefies) rapidly, producing toxic substances and putrefactive bacteria. The meat eater's intestinal tract, therefore, is very short, only three times the length of his body. He must rapidly digest meat and quickly eliminate the decaying waste products. The intestinal tract of the fruit and vegetable eater is twelve times the length of his body and provides the slow trip necessary for complete digestion of high-fiber, low-fat vegetable foods, which do not putrefy as rapidly. In fact, 5,000-year-old wheat found in the Pyramids germinated and sprouted when it was planted. Consider how nicely fruits and vegetables keep for days without refrigeration, then imagine eating some ground beef that has been sitting on your windowsill for four or five days.

Man the Mighty Hunter?

Contrary to belief, early man was not a mighty hunter. He was almost a complete vegetarian, eating only an occasional rodent encountered in his forage for food. Weapons needed for killing prey evolved late in man's history, and without them he was in no position to play a predatory role. He's one of the slowest mammals on earth, outrun by almost every other mammal except the three-toed sloth of South America (who even sleeps slowly). Indeed, even if man did catch something and kill it, he would be quickly run off by stronger, more competitive carnivores. Without a weapon, man is no match for a twenty-five-pound dog, or, much less, hungry meat eaters more his own size, like leopards, cheetahs, or wolves.

What the Experts Say

Almost all scientists and naturalists including Charles Darwin, who wrote on the theory of evolution, agree: Man's structure, internal and external, is designed for a diet of fruits, grains, and other high-fiber, high-carbohydrate vegetables.

Vaughn Bryant, Associate Professor of Anthropology at Texas A & M University, in his studies on cavemen, discovered their diet to be primarily vegetables (with an occasional grasshopper), very low in fat while high in carbohydrates and fiber. At the age of thirty-nine, and thirty pounds overweight, Professor Bryant went on a modified caveman diet by eliminating meat, eggs, butter, oil, and simple sugars. Instead he ate whole-grain bread, fruit, potatoes, rice, and a little fish. He lost the thirty pounds, kept it off, and noted a marked increase in his energy and well-being.

Back to Nature

Rarely does man voluntarily return to the primitive state, and only occasionally does it happen by accident. Remember that lone Japanese soldier who was isolated on an out-of-the-way island in the South Pacific and maintained a vigilant state of preparedness for thirty years after the end of World War II? He was forced to return to food gathering, living on edible leaves, fruits, and vegetables. When he was found and returned to civilization, doctors were amazed at his robust health. Close to sixty, he looked and tested out at not a day over forty. Imagine yourself on an island without tools or weapons or even fire. If there were fruits and vegetables around, they would instinctively be your first choice of food; a cat, on the other hand, would starve to death under the same circumstances if there were no smaller animals for it to eat.

A "Horror Story"

In California, before each Rose Bowl football game, a local restaurant has what it calls the "Steak Bowl." Each team is given a meal of all the steak they can eat, and usually there is a "humorous" report of an eighteen-year-old football player who "wins" by eating seven steaks and finishing off his meal with a quart of ice cream. I am horrified when I think of all that fatty, putrefying meat meandering slowly through his intestinal tract, silently loading his bloodstream with fat and cholesterol.

Are we the same species that put a man on the moon? While *complete* vegetarianism (using no animal products) is not necessary to obtain or maintain good health, no one can continue to eat the quantity of meat, eggs, cheese, and other high-fat, high-protein foods that Americans eat, and expect to stay healthy. It's like putting oil in your car's gas tank each morning and expecting it to run smoothly. If you are a big meat and potatoes man then you're likely to die like one—with clogged arteries, and a deteriorating heart.

Instinct versus Culture

The behavior and habits of a cat or dog are instinctive, and almost identical worldwide unless changed by man. As a result, animals of the same species generally eat the same kind of food regardless of where they live. Human beings, however, are not controlled by strong instincts, and have developed a myriad of cultures and customs that differ markedly from location to location. In short, we quickly learn behavior from our culture, "like father, like son," or "when in Rome, do as the Romans do."

And so it is that diet, as well as other cultural habits, follows definite guidelines from country to country. As children grow, their tastes are specifically governed and determined by habit and they "learn to like" their native food and crave it when hungry. While Americans are revolted at the thought of fried grasshoppers, they are a delicacy in other cultures.

When dietary patterns are being established, foods are never selected because they are healthy. More commonly, dietary patterns such as meat and milk consumption in this country are simply habits that spring up for no known reason. *After* they become habit *then* we look upon them as good.

Take for example the four basic food groups: Milk, Meat, Fruits and Vegetables, Breads and Cereals. This concept of balanced nutrition is taught in public schools. Not surprisingly, most Americans feel that this "balanced diet concept," in which milk and meat are undisputed stars, was passed down with the Ten Commandments, etched in stone. Yet, this ridiculous, disease-causing concept came into being in 1956. Our government was considering six basic food groups but instead narrowed it to four.

The milk and meat industries were overjoyed and "volunteered" to educate the public through the public school system. The biased brainwashing has been so effective that millions of Americans can't be convinced that heart disease, cancer, and other diseases are linked to those "nutritious" foodstuffs, milk and meat. Indeed, mothers across the country are absolutely terrified by the thought of not giving milk to their children. But where will they get their protein, and their calcium? they would ask. More on that in Chapter 10.

Whole cow's milk, in my opinion, is unfit for human consumption at any age, doing far more harm than good. It is unnecessary for calcium and protein or any other nutrient required for growth (all necessary nutrients can be obtained elsewhere) and it plays an integral role in the devastating diseases and early mortality rate of our culture. But milk and its products are so much a part of American life that it is listed as number one in the four basic food groups, despite studies showing whole milk to be dangerous.

Basically, we are locked into the high-fat diet by culture. The four basic food group concept, habit, and advertising all serve to perpetuate the beliefs of our culture. The fallacy of our beliefs about nutrition is apparent when we look at the nutritional habits of other cultures and compare.

Cultural Differences

There are three basic types of cultural diets: Western, Oriental, and underdeveloped. Western cultures include the Anglo-Saxon cultures of Russia, Europe, Scandinavia, England, the United States, and Canada. This diet emphasizes animal protein foods. In the Orient, which includes Japan, China, and other areas in the Far East, the diet is generally one of rice, vegetables, and some fish. The underdeveloped cultures sometimes called Third World countries depend on food of low-energy requirement for production. In other words, the food energy of grains is not used as animal food, but rather consumed by the culture itself. Most rural Mexicans, for example, eat very little meat because they can't afford it, although they do eat a lot of corn which in America is used to feed cattle. Other underdeveloped cultures follow the same patterns, existing as vegetarian food gatherers eating only limited amounts of meat or dairy products.

Percentage of Calories That Come from Fats, Carbohydrates, and Protein

In all cultures a variety of foods are eaten, and the only way to bring any order to the matter is to think in terms of the caloric composition of the diet as a whole. That is, foods consumed by a culture will contain a certain percentage of fat, protein, and carbohydrate calories.

The Western diet with its emphasis on meat and dairy products derives a lot of its calories from fat, while the Oriental and underdeveloped diets derive most of their calories from carbohydrates.

Notice that the percentage of protein calories in all three categories is more or less the same, but as the amount of *animal* source protein that is consumed increases, so does the death rate from heart disease.

Table IV-1 shows marked differences in the percentage of calories coming from carbohydrates and fat in the three cultures. These are also associated with marked differences in health problems. Namely, as the percentage of fat calories increases from culture to culture, so the number of deaths by heart disease increases as well.

TABLE IV-1

	FAT %	PROTEIN %	CARBOHYDRATE %
Western	43	12	45
Oriental	10	10	80
underdeveloped	10	10	80

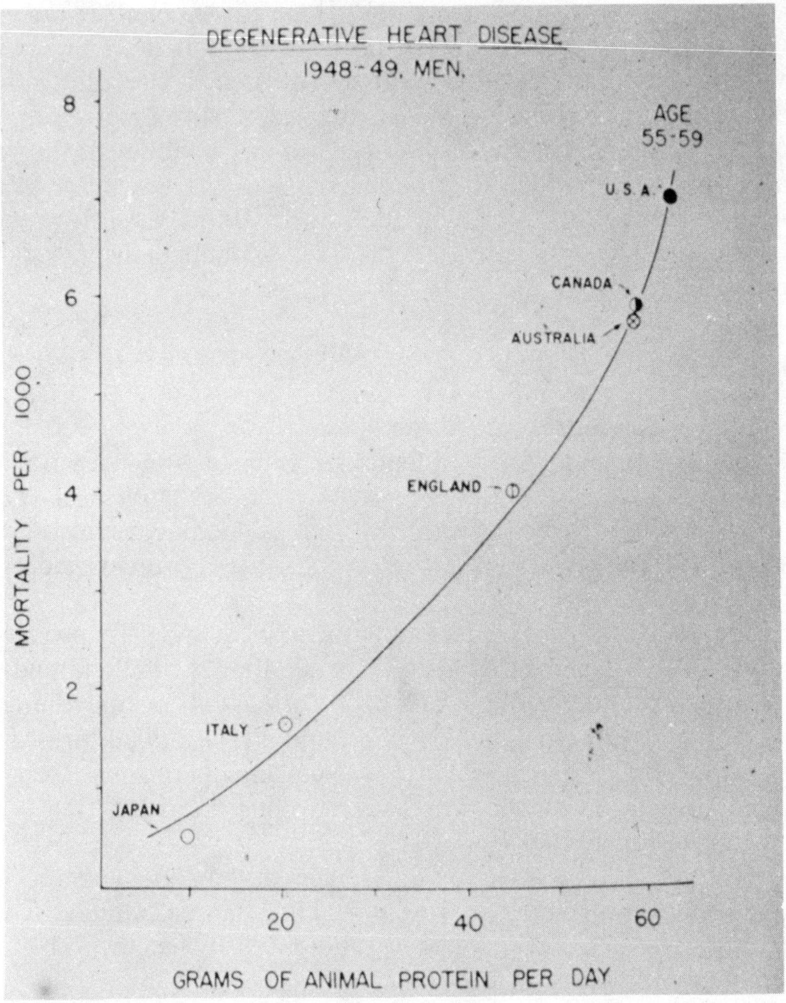

(Olsen, Robert E. "The effects of dietary protein, fat, and choline of the serum lipids and lipoproteins of the rat." *American Journal of Clinical Nutrition,* 6 (1958):111–118.)

Recording these observations is the job of epidemiologists whose findings often give us a big lead in trying to solve our heart disease problem. Epidemiological studies of twenty-five separate cultures demonstrated that those with diets containing only 10 to 12 percent fat calories had negligible, if any, heart disease. Second, when these cultures became acclimated to a culture with a diet high in fat calories, the scourge of heart disease quickly surfaced.

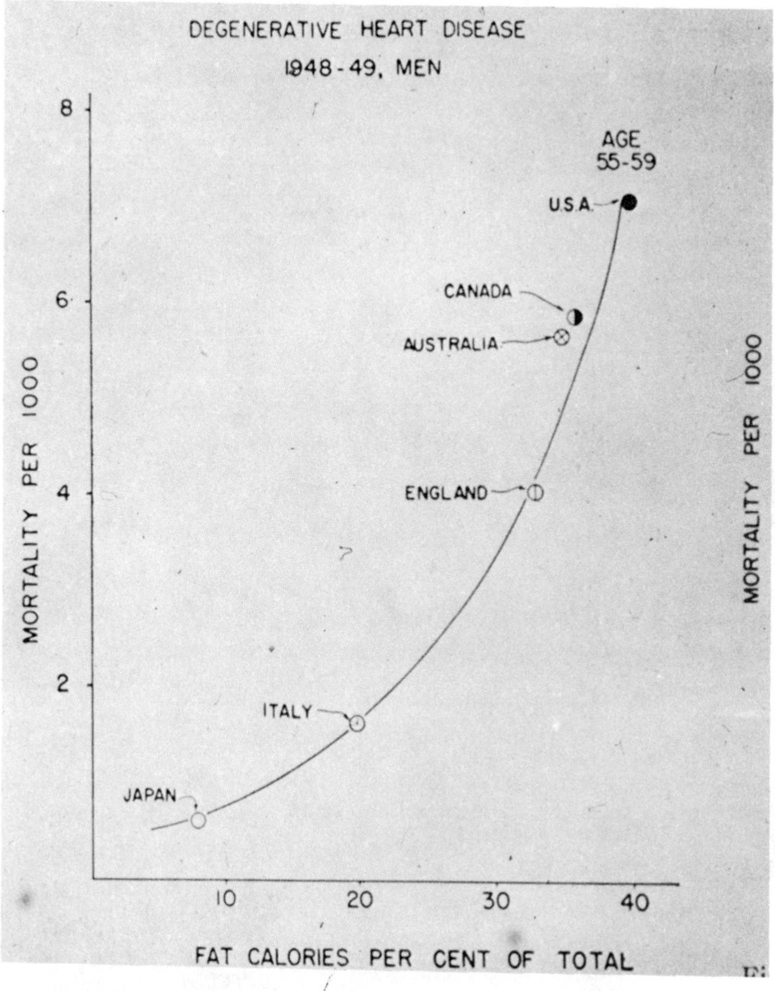

(Olsen, Robert E. "The effects of dietary protein, fat, and choline of the serum lipids and lipoproteins of the rat." ***American Journal of Clinical Nutrition,*** **6 (1958):111–118.)**

A case in point is South Africa, where the British settled and brought with them cream, butter, meat, and eggs. Heart disease rates among the British in South Africa are identical to those in England. In contrast, among the Bantu natives of South Africa, who exist on fruits and leafy vegetables, heart disease is almost nonexistent. The Nkana Nund Hospital serves both Bantus and Europeans in South Africa. During a five-year period in the 1950s not a single death due

1288 MEN AGED 40–49

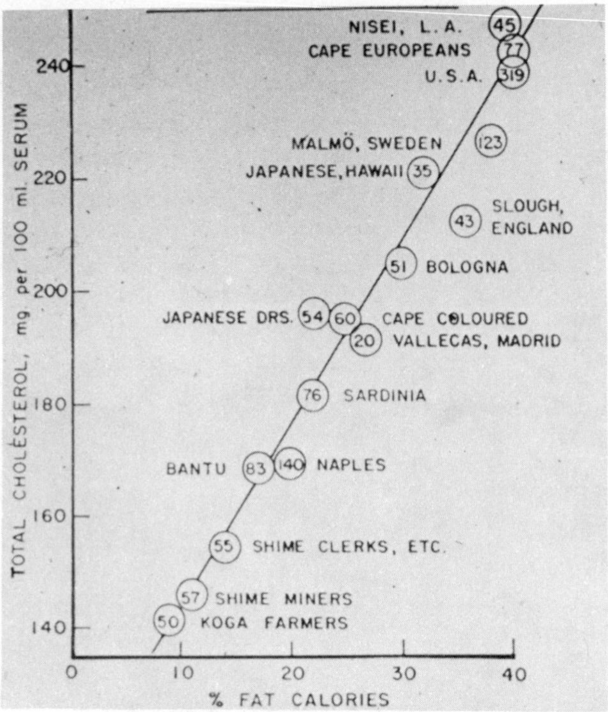

(Keys, Ancel. "Lessons to be learned from serum cholesterol level." *Annals of Internal Medicine,* 48 (1958):83.)

to heart disease was recorded among the Bantus, while twenty-three Europeans died from heart disease. And yet, only 10 percent of the hospital is utilized by the Europeans; 90 percent is utilized by the Bantus.

The Japanese Experience

The Japanese culture and their migration experience offer convincing evidence that a high-fat diet is the major cause of heart disease. On their traditional low-fat diet, only 10 percent of the calories come from fat and the Japanese have predictably low blood cholesterol levels, averaging 150. When Japanese migrate to Hawaii, they adopt the Polynesian dietary customs where the fat percentage of the calories is 30 percent. Predictably there is a rise in the blood cholesterol level to 200. Those Japanese who move to Los Angeles and adopt the high-fat (43 percent of the calories) diet there have blood cholesterol levels that reach 240, consistent with the American average at the time of the study.

Atherosclerosis, the treacherous problem of artery destruction, was measured in autopsies of Japanese men living in Japan, Hawaii, and the United States. In Japan no significant artery damage was found at any age, in Hawaii a moderate degree occurred, while in the United States the problem was severe and progressive. In fact, Japanese men living in America had more artery damage by the age of thirty than Japanese men living in Japan had by the age of seventy.

General epidemiological studies strongly implicate fat and high-cholesterol foods as the major factor in causing heart disease. There are a couple of apparent exceptions, which are not exceptions when studied.

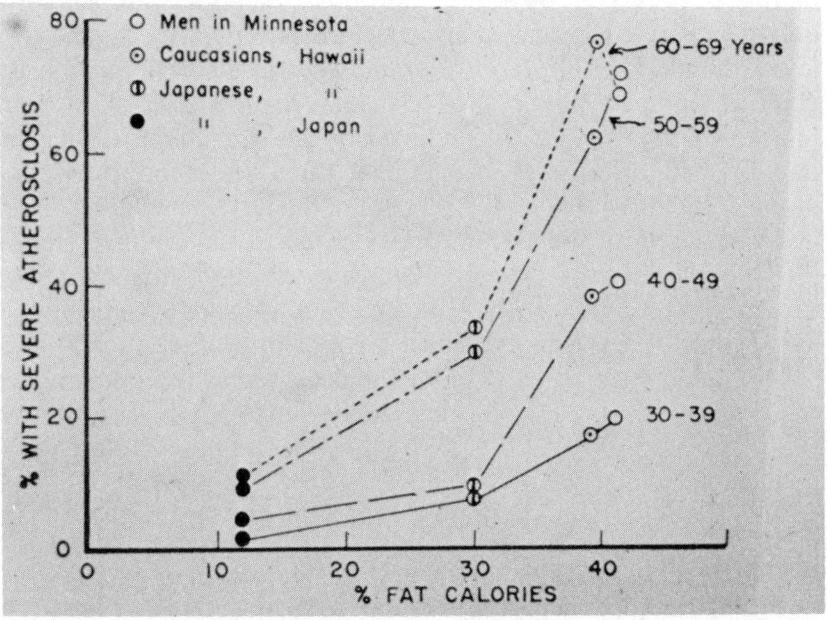

"Lessons to be learned from serum cholesterol level." (Keys, Ancel. *Annals of Internal Medicine*, 61 (1976):421.)

The Eskimo Experience

It has been known for some time that Eskimos, who consume a high-fat diet, have a low heart attack rate. This may reflect their adaptation to their harsh environment as they live in sub-zero temperatures with no heat. The average winter temperature is −37°F. The caloric energy necessary just to stay alive is enormous. As the Eskimo breathes this sub-zero air, it is heated and humidified by his body, which causes substantial loss of body heat. About 1,000 calories a day over the 2,000 calories needed for normal metabolism are required. With a diet that is inevitably frozen (as one would expect at −37°F), the Eskimo's body is further robbed of heat. His caloric requirement could be as high as 9,000 calories a day, and under these circumstances a high percentage of calorie-rich fat is probably necessary.

More importantly, however, the fat consumed by Eskimos comes exclusively from fish and marine mammals (seal and whale) and differs in composition from that consumed by Americans. These marine fats are very high in certain unsaturated fats and confer a degree of protection against atherosclerosis. First, they significantly lower the blood cholesterol level and elevate the HDL fractions of cholesterol (see Chapter 9) which alone reduces the risk of heart attacks among Eskimos. Second, marine fats are high in eicosapentaenoic acid, an unsaturated fat that thins the blood, protecting against clot formation. Only 1 percent of the fat consumed by Americans comes from fish and in order for Americans to duplicate the intake of the Eskimos, they would have to eat substantial quantities of mackerel or sardines. This change is not likely, or even desirable, as it would add to the excessive amount of protein already consumed, and cause an even more rapid degree of osteoporosis, or weakening of the bones. (This is discussed in Chapter 10.) However, supplementing a low-fat diet with some marine oils rich in eicosapentaenoic acid seems to be beneficial (see Chapter 13).

The Wandering Masai

Another people who seem to survive well on a high-fat diet are the Masai, a warlike cattle-herding people in Africa. Wandering from grazing ground to grazing ground with their cattle, the Masai men have their food supply with them on the hoof. They milk cows and also regularly bleed them, collecting the blood in a gourd. They mix the blood with milk and drink it. In spite of this high-fat concoction, they seem to have no heart disease.

The Masai paradox attracted the attention of an American researcher, George Mann of Vanderbilt University, who published a study about them in the 1960s showing that their electrocardiograms were normal and that heart attack was indeed rare among them. This study was gleefully pounced upon by the meat and dairy interests here and distributed to the media as proof that meat and milk don't plug the arteries.

But then George Mann went back to Africa and did autopsies on fifty Masai warriors who had died of various causes other than heart attack, causes that naturally happen among warriors and herdsmen. He found that their arteries were severely damaged with atherosclerosis—as badly as those of American men of the same age. But since Masai, walking with their cattle, get in about ten to twenty miles a day on foot, they had developed arteries twice the size of the average American's. Those big arteries, even though loaded with plaque, were delivering a full supply of blood and oxygen. The Masais' diet should have killed them, but their exercise saved them even though it did not prevent artery damage.

6

Fat: Inhibitor of Oxygen

You're an expert breather—you can even do it in your sleep. You started breathing at birth and have done it night and day ever since, with brief interruptions: 12 breaths a minute, 17,280 breaths a day, 6,307,200 a year. By the age of fifty you will have breathed 315,150,000 times. Why are you piling up this impressive record? To get oxygen.

The cardiovascular system, including the lungs, delivers oxygen to the millions of cells in your body. Without oxygen, life stops. Every bodily reaction depends on an uninterrupted flow of oxygen. In the simplest terms, life is the extraction of energy from food by a process that utilizes oxygen. As you read this book the complex brain processes of word recognition, association, memory, and memory storage are all dependent on large amounts of oxygen carried to the brain. Oxygen is needed all the time; the cardiovascular system never takes a vacation. If oxygen is cut off from the brain for only four minutes, irreversible brain damage occurs.

Red Blood Cells: Going Single File

Red blood cells have to go through small little narrow channels called capillaries, or else nothing will work in your body. The red blood cell is shaped like a shallow soup bowl and contains a special protein that carries oxygen. To get the oxygen into the body cells, the red cells go *single file* through the capillaries, the smallest blood vessels in the body which are five microns in diameter. A micron is one ten-thousandth of a centimeter—*small.* The red cells are a bit too large to go through the capillaries being about seven microns across. This might seem like poor planning but there is a purpose for it. It is in the capillaries that the red cells transfer oxygen to the stationary cells, taking on a load of carbon dioxide in exchange to be carried back to the lungs and exhaled. For this transfer or exchange the red cells have to cozy right up to the stationary cells, and that's why we have the snug fit of red cells in the capillaries. Red cells are elastic and can scrunch up a bit to get through the tiny tubes one by one, a little apart from each other. They appear to have a slight electromagnetic charge to repel each other. Therefore, red blood cells stay apart and flow smoothly through the capillaries. A fatty meal, however, ruins this.

How Fat Inhibits Oxygen Delivery

Fat is greasy to the touch; you know how it sticks to your fingers and has to be dissolved with soap or detergent to get it off. And it isn't processed to make it less sticky before it gets into the blood. Other nutrients get quite a processing. In the intestines carbohydrates are treated by enzymes to break them down into their simplest component, glucose. Proteins are similarly reduced to amino acids. The amino acids and glucose are carried directly to the liver, which stores them, alters them, and meters them out to the rest of the body as needed. Excess amino acids are broken down into urea and excreted in the urine.

Fats, however, are not actually broken down by digestion into their component parts but are emulsified by bile acids into small droplets called "chylomicrons." Unlike amino acids and glucose, which are carried directly to the liver by the bloodstream, fats are absorbed by the lymphatic system, a slow-moving auxiliary circulation to the blood system. The lymphatic system bypasses the liver and dumps the fat into the blood system at the level of the heart. From here, fat is pumped by the heart all over the body. Therefore, if you eat an excessive amount of fat, you will get an excessive amount in your bloodstream—unlike proteins and carbohydrates, whose blood levels are at least partially controlled by the liver.

In the bloodstream, fat gums up the circulation. Just as fat coats your fingers or a frying pan, it coats the red cells and makes them stick together like gummy poker chips. This is called "rouleaux formation," or "red-blood-cell aggregation."

As more and more fat enters the blood this clumping of red cells continues until there are masses of red cells that can't get through the capillaries. This causes a serious reduction of up to 30 percent in the oxygen supply to the tissues.

In the cardiovascular research laboratories at Wayne State University College of Medicine, Dr. Timothy Regan studied the way one high-fat meal impeded the supply of oxygen to the heart tissue. Healthy volunteers, people with no heart trouble, ate a fat-loaded meal. At peak levels of fat in the blood the oxygen uptake by the heart was reduced 20 percent. Dr. Regan then used heparin, a dangerous but commonly used blood-thinner, to clear the blood of fat. Oxygen uptake by the heart tissue went back to normal.

How Fats Bring on Angina

Angina pectoris, or chest pain, is the hallmark of heart disease and occurs because of corroded, blocked arteries. It comes on when the heart doesn't get enough oxygen in its tissue, and it has been compared to a scream by the heart for more oxygen. It is often—but not necessarily—brought on by physical activity. For some patients this might be shoveling snow; for others no more than trying to walk a few steps. Arteries to the heart that are dammed up with cholesterol deposits, and carrying fat-laden blood, can't deliver the oxygen needed for the increased activity.

Several years ago, Dr. Peter Kuo, from the University of Pennsylvania, gathered fourteen patients who had suffered from angina attacks for a rather rough but very illuminating experiment. In his office Dr. Kuo measured the fat in their blood and then gave each one of them a glass of cream to drink. He then measured the fat increase in their blood. Six of the fourteen patients had chest pains identical to those they experienced while climbing stairs or with

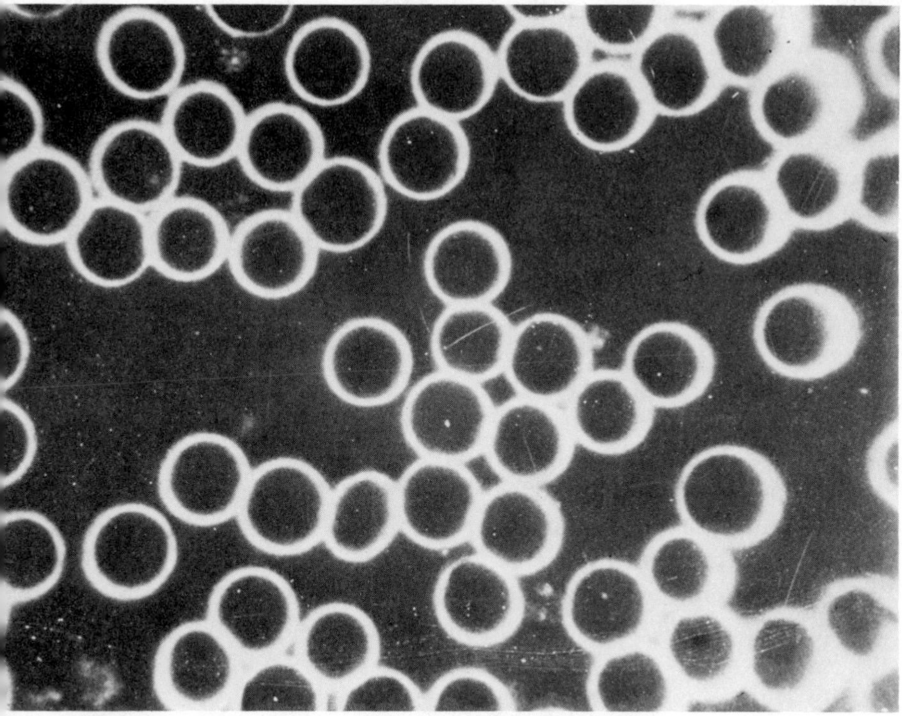

Blood cells normally space themselves and flow in single file.

After a high fat meal, blood cells clump together and can no longer flow through the capillaries.

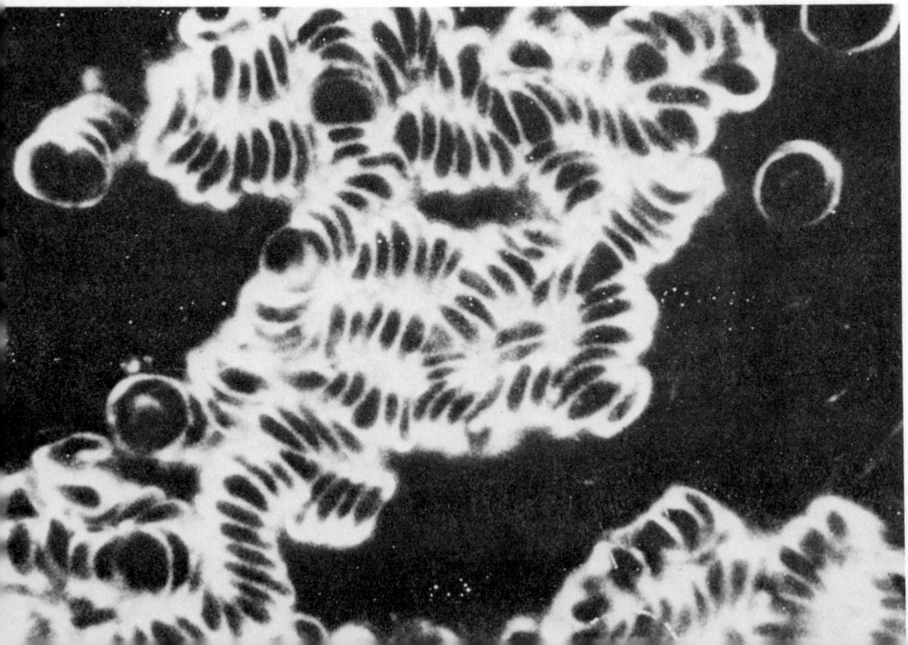

other kinds of exercise. Of these six patients, four showed definite changes on the electrocardiogram indicating that their hearts weren't getting enough oxygen. Dr. Kuo concluded that a high-fat meal "may exert a deleterious effect on the myocardium [heart muscle] in patients whose coronary circulation is already severely compromised by coronary artery disease. For this reason a low-fat diet may well be useful in the management of patients with angina pectoris, as a measure to help prevent their pain." The surprising study that showed that commonly eaten high-fat foods could, by themselves, bring on angina was published July 23, 1955, in the *Journal of the American Medical Association* (*JAMA*).

Taking the lead from Dr. Kuo, in 1957 Dr. Arthur Williams, of the Department of Medicine and Anatomy at the University of South Carolina, studied ten patients hospitalized with angina pectoris. He gave each one a hearty breakfast consisting of two fried eggs, a big slice of ham, toast with butter, and coffee with cream. (Sound familiar?) After the meal he observed small blood vessels in the whites of their eyes with a microscope and was able to watch the blood cells stick together and block the circulation. He concluded that his studies showed a ". . . definite relationship between the ingestion of fat, the agglutination of the blood, the stoppage of blood flow in the bulbar conjunctival vessels [in the eye], and, in those patients having the most severe agglutination of blood, the development of angina pectoris."

A Fat by Any Name. . .

A lot of people believe that animal fats in cheese, milk, eggs, and meat are dangerous but that vegetable fats such as safflower oil, peanut butter, corn oil, and margarine are safe. They are wrong. The red blood cells can't tell the difference. Vegetable fats cause clumping and oxygen deprivation. Dr. Meyer Friedman compared effects of animal fats like cream with vegetable fats like safflower oil on volunteer firemen. He found that both types caused red-cell clumping and, get this, the vegetable fats were worse in effect than the animal fats.

In 1965, in the *Journal of the American Medical Association,* Dr. Friedman concluded that ". . . the ingestion of unsaturated fats could lead to disaster as readily as ingestion of saturated fats. This possibility particularly looms as a potential danger, in view of the fact that the contemporary clinical fashion is not to advise the reduction of all fat in the diet, but only the substitution of unsaturated for saturated fats in the diet." If the name of Dr. Friedman is familiar to you it is probably because he wrote the big-selling book *Type A Behavior and Your Heart.*

You need *some* fat in your diet. But for good circulation you must keep intake of *all kinds* of fat very low.

The human system is not made for handling a big fat intake. Our high-fat diet plays a part in almost all the degenerative diseases—cancer, arthritis, diabetes, high blood pressure—as well as in heart disease. When fat deprives cells of adequate oxygen the cells start to degenerate and this is a prime cause of degenerative disease.

Next time you load a sandwich with mayonnaise, or open wide to bite into a greasy burger, think how that fat will ooze into your bloodstream, clump your red cells, and deprive your heart of oxygen.

7

The Process of Atherosclerosis

A man is as old as his arteries

Atherosclerosis, or "hardening of the arteries with plaque formation," is responsible for over 95 percent of the heart disease in this country. Actually, it is artery disease. The heart muscle is fine, but is "choked to death" by plugged arteries. It is this same atherosclerosis that brings on strokes, poor circulation in the legs, gangrene, and other dangerous, painful conditions.

Definition

Atherosclerosis and arteriosclerosis are sometimes used interchangeably, but the following definitions are more accurate:

ARTERIOSCLEROSIS (ahr teer ee o″ skle ro′sis)

Arteriosclerosis is the term used to describe the general process of damage and subsequent hardening of the major arteries. Arterio (artery) sclerosis (hardening, or scarring) results with almost any process that damages the arteries. Some relatively rare forms of arteriosclerosis are syphilis and specific collagen diseases like lupus erythematosus and polyarteritis nodosa.

ATHEROSCLEROSIS (ath″ur o″skle ro′sis)

Atherosclerosis is the specific process of fat and cholesterol damage and deposition (plaque build-up) in the artery. It is the most common form of artery damage and for the most part is synonymous with arteriosclerosis in American medical writing.

The Artery Lining

The large arteries in the body are muscular tubes lined with specialized cells called endothelial cells. These smooth cells give the artery an ideal surface for blood flow and serve as a barrier between the blood and muscle cells of the artery wall. These cells also produce a substance that thins blood and prevents blood clots, another substance that rapidly dissolves any small clots that may form, and a cell duplication inhibitor that prevents the underlying muscle cells from multiplying.

This layer of cells lining the arteries is much more specialized than anyone imagined fifteen years ago. The more we learn about it, the more we realize how important it is in protecting the artery from damage. And, like the watchmaker who loves and cares for fine watches, the more you know about the miracles of the healthy body and its sensitive, intricate systems, the more respect you have for it and the less likely you are to hurt yourself by eating the wrong foods. Loading your bloodstream with fatty hamburger or greasy sausage tears through this specialized cell layer like a fire in a paper mill, starting the deadly process of atherosclerosis. Human arteries were designed to stay open for a lifetime. Why not allow them to do so?

Atherosclerosis is a two-step process: First, the sensitive endothelial cells lining the artery are damaged, and second, elevated levels of fat and cholesterol circulating in the blood leak into the muscle layer of the artery. This irritates the muscle cells which actually engulf the cholesterol and start multiplying.

Step 1: Artery Lining Damaged

Oxygen Deprivation. The muscle cells, like all cells in the body, require a constant supply of oxygen. The outer two-thirds of the artery wall has its own blood vessels called "vaso-vasorum," or more literally, the "blood vessels to the blood vessels." The inner one-third has no blood vessels and is dependent upon diffusion of oxygen through the endothelial cell barrier. This dependence is one cause of the endothelial disruption which initiates the atherosclerotic process. When fat enters the blood in excessive amounts it causes the red blood cells to stick together. This reduces the oxygen supply throughout the body including the inner one-third of the artery wall. This damages some of the muscle cells and produces a generalized swelling of the artery wall. As you might imagine, this swelling pulls the endothelial cells apart in the same way the swelling of a bathroom floor would disrupt the tile covering.

Smoking and High Blood Pressure

Smoking and high blood pressure also disrupt this endothelial barrier. Smoking increases the carbon monoxide concentration in the blood which displaces oxygen from the red blood cells. Like too much fat in the blood, this lowers the amount of oxygen circulating and causes the irritation of the muscle wall which then swells. Even the so-called safe, low-tar cigarettes flood the lungs and bloodstream with carbon monoxide, lowering the oxygen supply. High blood pressure increases the shearing force of the circulating blood, thus mechanically injuring the sensitive endothelial cells and creating a defect in the barrier.

Dietary Cholesterol

Some studies have indicated that the cholesterol present in our diet not only elevates the blood cholesterol level leading to atherosclerosis (in the presence of a damaged endothelial lining), but also may damage the endothelial lining, thus doubling the damages. Dr. H. Imai has demonstrated that oxygenated molecules of cholesterol can cause severe artery damage in very small concentrations. Oxygenated cholesterol molecules are produced by exposure of cholesterol to oxygen and the tendency of cholesterol to undergo oxygenation was reported by the German scientist Dr. E. Schulze in 1904. These changes occur spontaneously with exposure to oxygen; add heat and the process is accelerated. Therefore, cooked meats, cooked eggs, and thin egg batters subjected to the intense heat of deep-frying are likely to contain substantial amounts of these highly toxic molecules.

Epidemiologic evidence of cholesterol's double-edged sword was recently published by Richard B. Shekelle in the *New England Journal of Medicine* in 1981. Nineteen hundred middle-aged men, working for the Western Electric Company, were studied for twenty years. Detailed information about their dietary habits was correlated and it was found that (1) those eating substantial amounts of cholesterol and saturated fat, as found in meats and dairy products, did indeed have elevated levels of blood cholesterol (an increased risk of heart disease) and (2) those eating substantial amounts of cholesterol foods had an increased risk of heart disease by some other means than the elevated level of blood cholesterol.

Surely other factors also disrupt the artery lining and allow cholesterol and fat to invade the artery wall. Inadequate intake of vitamin C could play a role. Vitamin C is essential for the maintenance of the body's connective tissue—the "glue" that holds the cell together. Even though enough of the vitamin may be present to prevent scurvy (a terminal deficiency of vitamin C), sub-optimal amounts may lead to weakening of the connective tissue bonding the endothelial cells, thus making them more vulnerable to disruption.

Step 2: Elevated Levels of Fat and Cholesterol

If blood cholesterol levels were to stay at 150 milligrams or less, endothelial injuries would repair themselves and be as good as new. With blood cholesterol levels above 150, however (the blood cholesterol level of the average American is a whopping 210), fat and cholesterol leak through the endothelial damage and into the muscle layer of the artery. This is like salt in a wound as cholesterol is extremely irritating to the muscle cells, which swell, multiply, and even engulf cholesterol particles. Once the process starts, this early plaque or cholesterol streaking continues if the blood cholesterol level stays high.

In the laboratory, rapid artery damage can be produced in certain animals by feeding them a high-fat, high-cholesterol diet and mechanically stripping away the endothelial cells of the large arteries. This is done by inserting a catheter into the artery, inflating

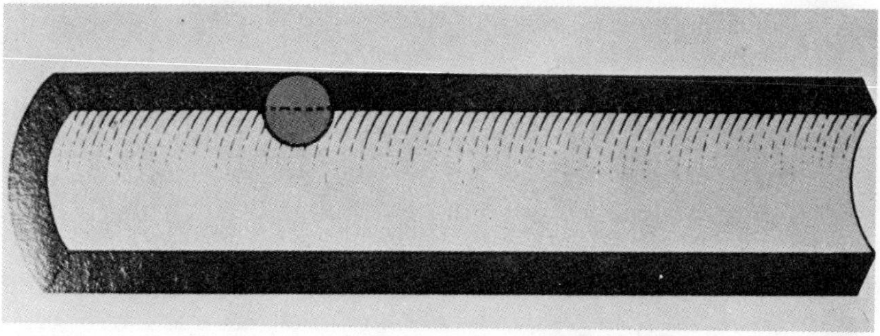

Initial event, the endothelial layer is damaged.

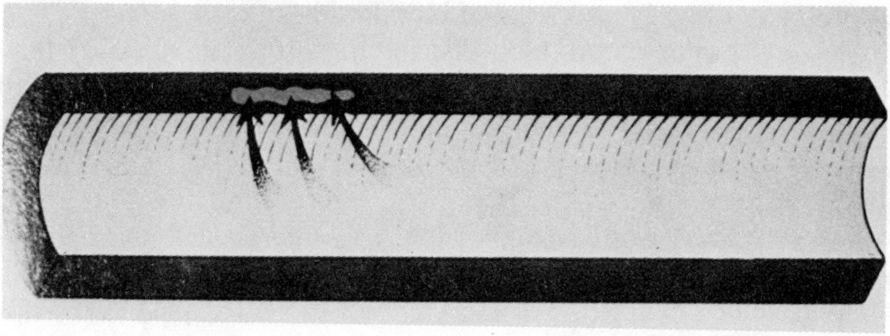

Then fat and cholesterol enter the muscle layer of the artery.

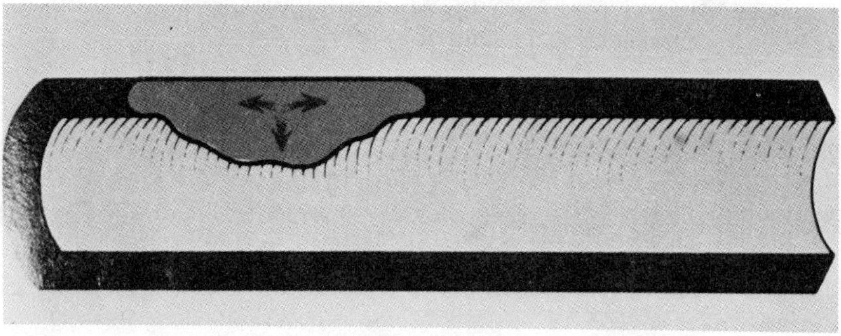

Destruction continues until the artery is closed.

a small balloon at the tip, then retracting the catheter. Dr. K.T. Lee, of the Department of Pathology at Albany Medical School, used this two-step procedure in fifteen pigs on a high-fat, high-cholesterol diet, causing catheter injury in coronary arteries to the heart. Rapid atherosclerosis ensued, and seven out of the fifteen pigs died suddenly with no warning in the same way humans would. The autopsies revealed massive atherosclerosis of the heart arteries and massive heart attacks.

An Unusual Case

I once met a thirty-seven-year-old woman at a seminar who told me that she had once had an aneurism from severe atherosclerosis of her abdominal aorta that had begun to swell like a balloon.

When she was thirty-six, this section of the aorta had to be replaced with a five-inch plastic graft. What interested me about her history was that this problem is rare in women at her age, as women seem to have protection during the child-bearing years. She then went on to tell me that two years before her surgery she was in an automobile accident and the steering wheel had rammed into her stomach. What surely had happened was that the crushing injury severely damaged the arterial lining, opening the door for atherosclerosis that later led to the aneurism. Of course, she was eating the same high-fat, high-cholesterol diet as everyone else.

Atherosclerosis—Silent but Deadly

Atherosclerosis is a silent killer. There are no nerve endings inside of the artery so we do not feel blood rushing through them or feel pain when the arteries begin to corrode. They can be totally destroyed before we realize anything is wrong. When you pick up a hot pan from the stove, you feel pain and quickly drop the pan. Without pain's sensations we would have no warning of danger. Remember, the first symptom of heart disease is often sudden death.

When people load their systems with such things as cheese omelets, fatty steaks, fatty salad dressings, and cigarette smoke, visualize the fat and cholesterol oozing into the bloodstream, clumping the red blood cells, blocking the capillaries, and cutting off the oxygen. Imagine the smooth glistening endothelial cells ripping apart because of the low oxygen tension, toxic cholesterol particles, and carbon monoxide. Next, the grease and cholesterol rush into the artery wall like medieval soldiers storming a castle. The sensitive muscle cells become irritated, swell, and begin to protrude into the lumen of the artery. The destruction process continues throughout the entire circulation, day in and day out, until it brings on a heart attack, stroke, or sudden death. Imagine all that destruction—and you don't feel a thing; in fact, you don't even realize that it is going on until, for many, it is too late.

Just because you can't see air
Doesn't mean it isn't there

8

High Blood Pressure

When the doctor takes your blood pressure he gets two readings, a high one and a low one, which he reads aloud as "one-twenty over eighty" and writes down as 120/80. The first number is the *systolic* or contraction reading and the second is the *diastolic* or expanding one.

The contractions and expansions are those of the heart—contracting to push blood into the arterial system and expanding to let blood flow into the heart from the veins.

When the heart contracts and pushes blood into the arteries the blood pressure goes up to the systolic reading. When it relaxes and expands, the blood pressure drops to the diastolic reading.

High blood pressure is more a condition than a disease, as there are gradations of severity. Generally, a blood pressure below 140/90 in the adult (children and teenagers should always have lower blood pressures than adults) is considered normal. Blood pressures from 140/90 to 160/110 are considered mild to moderate elevations, while any blood pressure above 160/110 is generally considered to be severe. Secondly, the blood pressure can vary significantly in a single individual. It is not unusual for a patient's blood pressure to be 145/95 on the first reading in a doctor's office; the traffic, concern generated by a trip to the doctor, and other factors are known to elevate the blood pressure. Fifteen minutes later, however, this elevated pressure will fall to a reading of 120/88. This is called "labile" high blood pressure and is known to affect a broad range of people. Therefore, the diagnosis of elevated blood pressure should not be made unless it is found to be elevated on several occasions and consistently so.

There is one area of confusion I would like to clear up: hypertension refers to high blood pressure, not to anxiety or emotional stress. True, anxiety and stress can, on occasion, elevate the blood pressure, but they do not always do this. For instance, someone who is under a lot of stress and feels anxious as well could very easily have a low blood pressure, while another individual could be very relaxed and under no stress with blood pressure of 160/110. A hypertensive individual is an individual with elevated blood pressures.

For most Americans with high blood pressure, an improper diet is the cause and a change in diet is the cure. Treating the condition with drugs often makes the condition worse, as I will explain shortly. The chief dietary substances affecting blood pressure are salt, fat, potassium, animal protein, and calcium.

Salt

Excess sodium in the system raises blood pressure, and nearly all the sodium in our diet comes from salt, otherwise called sodium chloride. Sodium attracts and holds water in the blood system, and it is the excess water that raises the blood pressure. Normally, drinking water will not by itself cause water retention; the kidneys, if functioning normally, can usually handle a water load, unless there is an excessive amount of sodium present that holds the water in your system.

The body needs some sodium but nowhere near what we generally eat. Most Americans load their food with salt because they are used to it, consuming ten to fifteen grams a day, which is twenty to thirty times the body's need. Many people get away with this without having high blood pressure, but for others the extra salt will add to a high-blood-pressure problem and increase the complications that go with it.

Several studies show that some hypertensive people who cut

down on salt intake will respond by lowering their blood pressure, but for many, simply restricting salt or sodium is just not enough. In fact, the whole concept of salt restriction as an effective method of lowering the blood pressure has recently come under fire. Dr. Norman Kaplan, professor of medicine, University of Texas, Southwest Medical School, points out that for many hypertensive individuals, the degree of salt restriction necessary to significantly reduce the blood pressure is so severe as to be impracticable. The amount of salt that is still present in most low-salt diets is so high as to still cause elevated blood pressure.

I am often frustrated when patients say, "Well, Doctor, I haven't used salt for years," as if this were enough to control the blood pressure, when in reality, it might be for them the least effective nutritional tool. For many patients and physicians, the fixation on salt restriction as the chief or only dietary tool available for lowering the blood pressure sets the stage for inadequate dietary control of blood pressure and leads to a host of dangerous drugs in order to bring the blood pressure down.

Let's now examine the other nutritional alterations that have an effect upon the blood pressure.

Dietary Fat

Salt is not the only nutrient known to increase blood pressure. Excessive dietary fat will as well. The mechanism for excessive amounts of fat causing elevated blood pressure is not completely understood, but one explanation is that fat causes the blood elements to stick together (as described in Chapter 6), so the heart has to work harder to push all that sludge around. I'm sure, however, that excessive fat alters a variety of the body's blood pressure controlling mechanisms.

When fat consumption is reduced, the blood pressure falls. Dr. Pekka Puska studied fifty-seven couples living in Northern Finland. This section of Northern Finland is noted for its high heart attack death rate, and has been the focus of several studies on the effects of various dietary changes in the hopes of isolating the factors that would reduce the heart attack death rate. In this study the couples were separated into three groups to determine what effect dietary changes had on the blood pressure. Group 1 reduced their fat intake from 40 percent of their calorie intake (similar to American intake of fat) to about 20 percent, with an increased percentage coming from vegetable fats. Group 2 reduced their salt intake by 50 percent, going from ten grams of salt daily to about five grams of salt daily, which is a substantial reduction. Group 3 made no change at all.

The only group that noted a drop in blood pressure was Group 1, the low-fat group. Systolic blood pressure dropped 8.9 mm of mercury and the diastolic dropped 6.6 mm of mercury. This drop was not due to weight loss or any factor other than the total fat reduction and the change in type of fat. From this study, reducing fat intake seems more powerful in lowering the blood pressure than even reducing the salt intake, as the no-salt group had no change in blood pressure. Dr. Puska concluded "salt intake reduction was ineffective in this trial. Thus changing dietary fat seems a promising method for the non-pharmacological treatment and prevention of hypertension."

Potassium

In addition to a high sodium (salt) intake, another cause of elevated blood pressure seems to be low potassium intake. In 1962, Dr. Naosuke Sasaki found that the average blood pressure of residents of two Northern Japanese towns was very different even though both consumed substantial amounts of salt. He found that the group with the lower blood pressure ate generous amounts of potassium found in apples that were a favorite of the town.

Graham A. MacGregor and colleagues at the Blood Pressure Unit, Department of Medicine, Charing Cross Hospital Medical School, London, England, demonstrated that adding 2.3 grams of potassium to a group of twenty-three hypertensive individuals reduced their mean blood pressure eight millimeters of mercury. They concluded that

> dietary alterations of sodium and potassium intake may obviate the need for drug treatment in many patients with essential hypertension and it may also improve the efficacy of drugs in those patients in whom dietary measures alone are insufficient.

> A moderate increase in potassium intake . . . could be achieved with a potassium-base salt substitute which could be added either in cooking or at the table and by a moderate increase in fresh fruit and vegetable consumption . . . . This study provides strong evidence of a blood pressure–lowering effect of a lacto ovo vegetarian diet in healthy normal omnivorous subject. These blood pressure changes were reversible within 5–6 weeks of returning to an omnivorous diet.

Animal Protein

Even when there's no difference in the consumption of salt, fat, or potassium, the type of protein consumed has an effect on blood pressure. Animal protein tends to increase blood pressure while vegetable protein tends to decrease blood pressure. Dr. Frank Sacks reported that simply substituting animal protein in the diet of vegetarians caused a significant increase in blood pressure. Dr. Ian Rouse, of the Department of Medicine, University of Western Australia, found that switching a group of omnivores to a lacto-ovovegetarian diet caused a significant drop in blood pressure that was not related to sodium or potassium intake.

Calcium

Calcium recently burst on the national scene as an important nutrient in controlling high blood pressure. An interesting study published by David A. McCarron, Associate Professor of Medicine of the Oregon Hypertension Program in Portland, Oregon, demonstrated that reduced daily calcium intake is associated with high blood pressure. Using a computer he assessed certain nutrient intakes in 10,372 individuals ranging in age from eighteen to seventy-four years. These people denied any history of high blood pressure or any intentional modification of their diet. He found that significant decreased consumption of calcium, potassium, vitamin A, and vitamin E were associated with increases in high blood pressure. Low calcium intake was the most consistent factor in hypertensive individuals. In his study group those individuals who had the higher calcium intake had the lowest blood pressure.

Almost simultaneous with this epidemiological report of large groups of people came a study by Dr. Lawrence Resnick, from Cornell University. In twenty-six patients with mild high blood pressure, two grams of calcium carbonate in divided doses caused the blood pressure to fall in sixteen of the twenty-six patients. In the overall group, the blood pressure fell from 161/94 to 154/89, a 5-point decrease in the important diastolic (second measurement) pressure. However, sixteen of the twenty-six patients experienced a drop of 10 points or more in the diastolic pressure.

He also found beneficial changes in the way the individuals handled sodium. Taken as a whole, these two studies mentioned above, as well as the other studies showing potassium, fat, and other nutrients to have an effect on blood pressure, usher in a whole new set of assumptions about high blood pressure. As physicians we can no longer advise our patients to eliminate dietary salt and assume that this is the only nutritional tool available. High blood pressure should be treated with a variety of nutritional tools and dietary modifications.

**Case history: The hypertensive pilot.* Frank M. had a problem. He was a fifty-four-year-old airline pilot, and was sure to lose his license. Commercial pilots may not have high blood pressure or be on medication for it and continue to fly. Frank checked into the Institute three weeks before his Federal Aeronautics Administration (FAA) physical exam with a blood pressure of 225/115. He had to get it down fast without medication, so we altered the diet even more radically than we usually do. He was allowed to eat nothing but fresh fruits, raw vegetables, and brown rice. This speeded up the blood-pressure-lowering capability of our program by drastically lowering salt, fat, and animal protein while just as dramatically raising the potassium. Frank checked out of the Institute in twelve days with a blood pressure of 130/84, on no medications. One week later he passed his FAA physical with a blood pressure of 140/82. Almost three years later Frank is still flying, and taking care of himself by following the more-diversified program in this book; he had a blood pressure of 120/75—on no medication.

Dangers of the Drug Treatment

Voluminous research shows that dietary changes could eliminate high blood pressure in many hypertensive patients. In spite of that, the routine approach for many M.D.'s is to immediately start a patient on drugs before, and usually without any recommendation for, a dietary change. The dangerous side effects of the drugs used make this approach, in my opinion, often more harmful to the patient than beneficial.

Diuretics, used to promote water elimination, are the drugs most commonly used. For instance, the thiazide diuretics such as Dyazide, Hydrodiuril, and Diuril have been shown to cause irregular heart rhythms. Dr. P.K. Whelton, who heads the British Medical Research Council trial of therapy, found that 33 percent of patients taking thiazide preparations had five irregular heartbeats an hour in the daytime, and 20 percent of the whole group had them at night as well. Of the control group, who were taking only a placebo, only 20 percent of them had irregular heartbeats in the daytime and 9 percent at night.

Irregular heartbeats often result when the blood potassium was reduced below normal. This occurs regularly in 10 to 15 percent of patients taking thiazide diuretics. Dr. Brian Holland studied twenty-one patients who had thiazide-induced low blood potassium levels and found that seven of them (33 percent) developed irregular rhythms.

In addition to causing an irregular heartbeat, thiazide diuretics have adverse effects on the metabolism. They have long been known to cause elevations of both the blood sugar and uric acid; the drugs will exacerbate or even cause diabetes, gout, or both. Thiazides also raise the blood cholesterol and triglycerides, which would negate their value as blood-pressure-lowering agents. High blood pressure is one of the three major risk factors for heart disease and strokes, elevated cholesterol and smoking being the other two. As Dr. Richard H. Grimm, of the Department of Medicine at the University of Minnesota Medical School, put it:

> An increase in serum total cholesterol and low-density lipoprotein fraction may increase coronary heart disease in pa-

> tients treated with diuretics. This has special implication in hypertensive persons already at excess risk for atherosclerosis and coronary heart disease. Even a small average increase in these lipid fractions would have considerable public health import because of the millions taking these drugs. Consequently, it is important to clarify the relation between diuretics and blood lipid changes in a controlled trial.

Dr. Grimm's study was published in 1981 in the *Annals of Internal Medicine.* In that study, sixty men with mild high blood pressure—defined as diastolic pressure between 90 and 105—were divided into groups receiving one of two commonly used diuretics or a placebo. Of those taking hydrochlorothiazide (the most commonly used thiazide) the cholesterol increased an average of 14.8 mg. Of those taking chlorthalidone (another thiazide) the cholesterol increase was 18.8 mg. Triglycerides also increased, as did the uric acid, with both thiazide diuretics. Dr. Grimm concluded that

> . . . the results of this study clearly show an adverse lipid metabolic affect for commonly used anti-hypertensive agents, the thiazide group of diuretics, known previously to affect glucose and uric acid mechanisms. This finding underscores the importance of continued research in the application of non-pharmacological means to lower blood pressure (weight loss, exercise and dietary sodium restriction), both as an adjunct to drugs and as primary treatment in a hygienic, preventive approach to blood pressure lowering.

Dr. Jan Drayen, of the University of California-Irvine College of Medicine, has found that many patients now receiving thiazide diuretics might be "non-responders," patients in whom the diuretics no longer bring down the blood pressure. Of fifty patients given thiazides, he found that 25 to 50 percent were non-responders. The reasons for the failure are probably due to the alteration of the other blood-pressure agents produced by the body in response to the thiazide diuretic. For instance, as the diuretic lowers the blood pressure by causing sodium excretion, the body counters by increasing the production of two hormones, renin and aldosterone, which decrease sodium loss. Result: increased blood pressure. The net result is that for many patients, these diuretics have no effect on the blood pressure, yet the patients suffer the significant dangers of the drugs themselves. And very often, other drugs are added to bring down the blood pressure.

I have concentrated on the thiazide diuretics because in my opinion they are a clear and present danger for those taking them—with no strong evidence of benefit. In an interview with *Medical Tribune* in 1984, Dr. David McCarron, from the University of Oregon, pointed out that "in terms of laboratory tests, there is no single agent that the physician can prescribe that has more adverse effect than a thiazide diuretic."

They are without doubt the most commonly prescribed drugs for men and women with mild or moderate elevation of blood pressure, representing usually the first drug that is prescribed. If blood-pressure control is not achieved, then other medications are usually added to the diuretic therapy. In fact, the thiazide diuretics have become so commonly used that drug companies recently have come out with combinations of thiazide diuretics added to other hypertensive medications. Examples: Indride (Inderal plus thiazide); Tomolide (Tenormin plus thiazide); Minizide (Minipress plus thiazide).

No one study has produced convincing evidence that using thiazide diuretics reduces the death rate of the mildly hypertensive patient with blood pressures ranging from 140/90 to 160/100. In fact, a large-scale government-funded study called the Multiple Risk Factor Intervention Trial (MRFIT) found that the mortality rate was actually higher in a group of hypertensive patients that received aggressive treatment compared to a group of hypertensive patients that received no treatment or less aggressive approaches. Another study by Dr. Anders Helgeland, of Oslo, Norway, demonstrated that the incidence of sudden death among patients with mild hypertension who were treated with hydrochlorothiazide was three times that of the control group not treated with the drug.

A particularly alarming study was published by Dr. Gary Cutter, head of the biometry division and associate professor of biostatistics at the University of Alabama. In a series of 5,000 patients who had undergone a cardiac catheterization and angiogram during the years 1970 to 1978 and who had been followed annually, those taking diuretics had a 1.4 times greater death rate than those not taking diuretics. Also, those taking diuretics had 1.5 times greater risk of death from cardiac disease. He did not specify the type of diuretic that was utilized, but the thiazide diuretics are by far the more commonly used.

Considering all the potential harm of thiazide diuretics, a few physicians are now sounding the alarm. Dr. Edward D. Freis, of the Veterans Administration Medical Center in Washington, D.C., published an editorial in the *New England Journal of Medicine* entitled, "Should Mild Hypertension Be Treated?" In it he challenged the concept of drug therapy for mildly hypertensive patients, pointing out that treatment could be worse than the disease.

My concern with use of the thiazide diuretics is that even after further studies indicate their definite and potential harm, they will still be utilized by many physicians for years to come because they have been so much a part of medical practice. Thiazide diuretics have been in use for over thirty years, with most physicians believing that they were safe and necessary. Hopefully, this book will stimulate appropriated interest in using diet changes as a first step in treating people with high blood pressure. I am convinced that for the overwhelming majority of people with mild to moderate elevations in blood pressure, this program is all that would be necessary. It certainly, in my opinion, should be used in all hypertensive patients to cut down on the requirements for medications.

9

The Cholesterol Confusion

I thought of calling this chapter The Cholesterol Controversy, but in reality there is very little controversy left. The top scientists are in accord that dietary cholesterol is bad for you and a major cause of cardiovascular disease in this country. However, because Americans are so used to high-fat, high-cholesterol foods, and because there is a substantial food lobby that opposes any dietary change, many people are still confused on the issues.

Here are some general questions which we want to address in this chapter.

1. What effect does diet have on the blood cholesterol level?
2. Elevated blood cholesterol levels—what risk do they represent in the development of heart disease?
3. Cholesterol is needed for the production of sex hormones, adrenal hormones, and for the assimilation of Vitamin D. Does this mean that we need to eat cholesterol?
4. Our bodies do indeed make approximately ten times the amount of cholesterol that we would eat, even on a high-cholesterol diet. Therefore, how can eating this relatively small amount of cholesterol create such a problem?
5. My physician told me that my blood cholesterol level was within the normal range, or average. Does this mean that I am not at risk for developing heart disease?

6. What is more important, the total cholesterol level in the blood, or the HDL cholesterol?
7. I have heard that egg yolks contain lecithin, which protects from the cholesterol that it also contains. Is this true?

Now the facts.

What Is Cholesterol?

Cholesterol itself is not a fat but a waxy noncaloric substance carried in the bloodstream along with fat. It is essential to life as it is necessary for the production of sex hormones and adrenal hormones, as well as vitamin D. It is also necessary for the synthesis of bile necessary for digestion.

The body produces all of the cholesterol it needs for these functions, and if you did not eat any cholesterol, your blood level would stay at the very safe 150 mg (average) percent range. There is never a need to eat any cholesterol; cholesterol is not a nutrient and ingestion of it can only harm you.

There is widespread belief that if you cut down on cholesterol foods your body will simply manufacture more cholesterol to keep the blood level the same. This is just not true. Almost all of the studies show that the body makes cholesterol at a more or less set rate and there is very little if any feedback control by diet. This means that the cholesterol you eat is simply added to the bloodstream thus elevating the cholesterol level. Secondly, the cholesterol level can be lowered in almost everyone by significant dietary changes.

Dietary Cholesterol

Cholesterol is present in all foods of animal origin, and is absent in all vegetable foods. Even if an animal-derived food is low in fat, such as fish or chicken, it still contains substantial amounts of cholesterol, while even very high vegetable-fat foods, such as corn oil, margarine, and peanut butter, contain no cholesterol. However, it is important to understand that good health requires reduction of all forms of fat, both animal and vegetable, as well as the cholesterol which is present only in animal-derived foods.

We can lump the cholesterol-laden animal foods into groups. The first group is the animal flesh foods, consisting of fish, chicken, and meat which all contain about 20 to 25 mg of cholesterol per ounce. The second group is shellfish, including shrimp, crab, and lobster, which have significantly higher concentrations of cholesterol, 50 to 75 mg per ounce. The third group is the organ meats such as liver, kidneys, brain, and sweetbreads which contain 70 to 120 mg of cholesterol per ounce. These foods may vary in fat content; shrimp, for instance, is relatively low in fat compared to steak which is very high in fat.

The king of cholesterol-laden foods deserving a group by itself is the egg. A single egg contains 275 mg of cholesterol, all of it found in the egg yolk. Eggs are the major source of cholesterol in the American diet, and contribute 30 to 55 percent of the cholesterol that Americans eat. We cannot overemphasize the contribution egg yolks make to cholesterol intake. For instance, naturally healthy low-fat, low-cholesterol foods such as pancakes and breads become dangerously high in cholesterol when egg yolks are added. The usual three-egg omelet contains 825 mg of cholesterol which is more cholesterol than two pounds of hamburger meat. Therefore, to suggest that you cut down on high-cholesterol foods and eat only a few eggs per week is like telling an alcoholic to cut down on his drinking and have only seven drinks a day! Because of their high concentration of cholesterol, egg yolks cannot and should not be part of any diet to lower the blood cholesterol level. Egg whites, however, are void of cholesterol and fat and provide the high-quality, balanced protein so valuable in eggs, and can be part of any diet.

Dietary Cholesterol and the Blood Level

When you eat cholesterol, it enters the body and adds to the blood cholesterol level, elevating it from the safe range of 150 to the very high ranges found in the American population. Numerous studies, as far back as the late '50s and early '60s, demonstrated that cholesterol and fat (primarily saturated fat found in animal foods) markedly elevate the blood level. Dr. William E. Connor, from the Department of Internal Medicine at the University of Iowa College of Medicine, studied six volunteers who went on a cholesterol-free diet and experienced a marked drop in their blood cholesterol level, from 249 mg percent to 191 mg percent. At the end of four weeks they were put on egg yolks in varying amounts and the blood cholesterol level shot up immediately from 191 mg percent to 260 mg percent—higher than the original average level. Back on the cholesterol-free diet, the blood level dropped down from 260 to 206, only to rise again to 224 when crystalline cholesterol was added to the food.

He concluded that "the addition of dietary cholesterol in the form of egg yolk caused a significant increase and concentration of cholesterol in the blood."

The Saturation Phenomenon

In most studies done on the effect of dietary cholesterol on the blood cholesterol level, an initial two to three weeks of low cholesterol foods invariably lowers the original blood cholesterol level. Then as dietary cholesterol is added to the diet, the blood level again elevates an average of 20 to 40 percent. However, after eating about 600 to 750 mg of dietary cholesterol (that found in approximately $2\frac{1}{2}$ eggs) there is no further elevation in the blood level. This is the saturation point, and reflects the inability of the intestinal tract to absorb more than 600 to 750 mg of cholesterol over a twenty-four-hour period. Additional intake of high-cholesterol foods does not continue to elevate the blood level but still poses a danger as these very large amounts of cholesterol pass through the colon and represent, according to many studies, a distinct cancer risk. (As you may have read, high-fat, high-cholesterol foods are now firmly established as increasing the risk of various cancers.)

Dr. J.M.R. Beveridge, of Queens University in Kingston, Ontario, studied ninety-three college students at the University Center. An initial fat-free, cholesterol-free diet produced a marked drop in their average blood cholesterol level, from 201 to 146 in only eight days. After stabilizing on the no-cholesterol diet, cholesterol foods were returned, starting with small amounts. Dr. Beveridge found that as little as 13 mg of cholesterol, or the amount of cholesterol found in one-half ounce of hamburger, caused a slight, but measurable, increase in the blood cholesterol level. The blood level continued to rise with each increase of cholesterol in the diet until the dietary cholesterol reached 600 to 700 mg. Again, above this level of dietary intake no further increase in the blood level was noted, but the volunteers had elevated their blood level back to the original 201. Saturation had occurred which meant that an additional three to four, or even five eggs containing thousands of milligrams of cholesterol would not have a measurable effect on the blood level.

This saturation phenomenon is analogous to pouring the contents of a one-quart pitcher into an eight-ounce glass. The first several ounces have an obvious effect on the water level in the glass. However, continued pouring would result in only eight ounces in the glass, plus a mess. If you eat the typical American diet, which contains eggs, fatty meats, and milk, you average 600 to 750 mg of cholesterol a day. Therefore, the elevating effect of cholesterol on your blood level has already maximized—it cannot go any higher. Your glass is full. But your cholesterol level is in the very dangerous range and is 50 to 100 points higher than it would be if you were eating safer low-fat, low-cholesterol foods.

Elevated Blood Cholesterol and Heart Attacks

The average American adult cholesterol level, because of the high-fat, high-cholesterol diet, is about 210 and is dangerously high. Therefore the national method of dying is heart disease. As early as 1958 Dr. Ancel Keys, Professor Emeritus at the Laboratory of Physiological Hygiene, at the University of Minnesota, stated that "one effect of our kind of high fat diet is hypercholesterolemia [elevated blood cholesterol], and this is so universal among us that our so-called cholesterol norms are simply standard for pre-clinical coronary disease [heart disease]. Hypercholesterolemia simply promotes atherosclerosis." Dr. Robert Maley, from the National Heart, Lung, and Blood Institute, recently pointed out that ". . . elevated plasma cholesterol is almost universally recognized as a risk factor in both the development of atherosclerosis and coronary heart disease." Dr. Maley's observation is in agreement with that of Dr. Robert Levy, director of the National Institute of Health, who stated that "high serum cholesterol levels, along with cigarette smoking, high blood pressure, have been clearly established as the major risk for coronary heart disease . . . the higher the cholesterol, the greater the risk." This dangerous and unequivocal relationship between elevated blood cholesterol levels and heart disease has been upheld in twenty-one out of twenty-one worldwide studies. Those with elevated blood cholesterol levels are at the greatest risk of heart attack.

The big question: What constitutes elevated blood levels? Answer: Any blood level above 150. Dr. Robert Wissler, of the University of Chicago, and Dr. William Castelli, a director of the Framingham studies, point out that a cholesterol level of 150 or lower almost guarantees immunity from heart disease. In 5,000 men followed for over twenty-five years in the Framingham, Massachusetts, studies, those with blood cholesterol levels of 150 or lower have yet to have a heart attack or die from heart disease.

As the blood level rises, atherosclerosis occurs, and the higher the level the more the risk of a heart attack. This means that the man with a blood cholesterol level of 190 does have a measurable risk of a heart attack but his risk is much lower (about one-fifth) than the man with the blood cholesterol level of 260.

"Normal" Is Deadly

Most laboratories issue a graph indicating that the "normal range" for cholesterol is between 150 to 300. This is insane! Within this so-called normal range, a man with a cholesterol level at the upper end has an infinitely greater risk of dying suddenly from a heart attack than does a man with a cholesterol level at the lower end. In fact, the average blood cholesterol level in this country, as mentioned, is a whopping 210, which as we all know puts the average American right in the middle of an epidemic. This is one time you don't want to be normal.

Take for example the average blood cholesterol level of the men or women lying in the coronary care unit having just suffered a heart attack. It is about 220—well within the so-called normal range. This means that contained in those heart attack victims with an average of 220 blood cholesterol level are some with elevated levels in the 260 to 290 range, as well as others with low levels in the 180 to 200 range. All of these patients are well within what is considered to be normal or okay.

An editorial by Irving S. Wright, in the *Journal of the American Medical Association* in July, 1976, concluded that accepting the current average cholesterol readings as normal is

> . . . both confusing to many physicians and detrimental to the proper care of patients. It has provided an excuse for avoiding the discipline necessary for prevention and treatment programs. The physician who accepts such laboratory "normals" is not acting on the basis of the best scientific criteria, and his patient may be misguided in planning his dietary pattern.

Planned Confusion—the Saturation Hoax

If diet elevates everyone's blood cholesterol to dangerous levels, where did I read that diet had no effect upon the blood level?

Several studies have appeared over the last few years that seem to show that cholesterol in food has little effect on the blood cholesterol level. Most of these studies, however, have been inaccurately reported by the lay press, giving false impression. For instance, one such study was done by Dr. Rosylyn Alfin-Slater, a research scientist at UCLA. She recruited a group of volunteers and studied the effect of adding an egg to their customary diets. After several weeks on the extra egg, she measured her volunteers' blood cholesterol level and found no change. But you must remember that her volunteers were on the general American diet, which is loaded in saturated fat and cholesterol (600 to 700 milligrams per day), and therefore would be saturated with dietary cholesterol. Therefore, one would predict that the extra egg would have no significant effect upon their blood cholesterol level, which was already elevated. In fact, Dr. Alfin-Slater stated in her original publication that "after certain levels of intake of cholesterol in the diet, further increases in the dietary cholesterol have little effect on the blood level. Therefore, since many of the subjects were already eating eggs as part of their normal diet, they would not be expected to show a marked increase in plasma cholesterol level."

Several months later a feature article appeared in the *Los Angeles Times* headlined, "New Study Explores Nutrition—Cholesterol Links Are Questioned." In this article Dr. Alfin-Slater was asked if the cholesterol people eat determines their levels of blood cholesterol. Her response to the question was "No correlation," but the article failed to mention that all of the volunteers in her study were already saturated with dietary cholesterol, so the net result of this reporting of the study was confusing.

A similar study was published by Margaret Flynn, Ph.D., at the University of Missouri. She also added an extra egg to the diet of a group of volunteers already eating substantial amounts of cholesterol. She then reported the predictable, no change in blood cholesterol level, as these volunteers also had reached the saturation point before the extra egg was added to their diet. This particular study received wide publicity in the *National Enquirer* with a headline banner that read, "Ten Year Study Proves Diet Not Linked to Dangerously High Levels of Cholesterol." The article went on to state inaccurately that Flynn's study had shown that "diet is not linked to cholesterol levels in the body, so an average person could eat meat, eggs, and other foods without fear of increasing the risk of heart disease." It is obvious that both the *Los Angeles Times* and the *National Enquirer* have not completely grasped the issue, contributing to the confusion about the effect of the cholesterol in our food on the circulating cholesterol in our blood.

In a more recent study published by Dr. Frank Sacks of Brigham and Women's Hospital in Boston, an extra egg to the diet was shown to be very dangerous indeed. His volunteers were seventeen vegetarian college students who consumed limited amounts of dairy products that brought their cholesterol intake per day to only 100 milligrams. Dr. Sacks added one large egg to their diet in the form of a muffin prepared with the egg. This increased their cholesterol intake per day to 400 milligrams and caused a 12-percent elevation in their circulating LDL cholesterol levels. As we will discuss, this fraction—the LDL—is the most dangerous fraction of cholesterol and a 12-percent rise would increase the risk for developing heart disease by over 25 percent—all of this from just one egg.

In an interview with Associated Press about his study, Dr. Sacks said, "What I wanted to try to hammer home in that paper was that conventional guidelines for lowering the cholesterol intake stopped too soon." Indeed, if you want protection from heart disease, one egg a day is a disaster. If you already have heart disease, that extra egg simply perpetuates the disaster.

What the Experts Really Think

Is there a controversy on the cholesterol issue or is it something the meat and dairy industries have fabricated to protect their interests? Dr. Kaare Norum, Professor of Nutrition at the University of Norway, was concerned with what he viewed as confusion on some relatively unconfusing relationships. He sent a questionnaire to 211 of the world's top scientists doing research in the area of fat and atherosclerosis. The three main questions and responses were:

> **1.** Do you think there is a connection between diet and the development of coronary heart disease?
> 188 said yes, 1 said no, 4 were uncertain; a 97 percent "Yes" response.
> **2.** Do you think there is a connection between diet and plasma lipoprotein level [blood cholesterol level]?
> 189 said yes, 2 said no, 2 were uncertain. A 98 percent affirmative response.
> **3.** Do you think there is a connection between plasma cholesterol and the development of coronary heart disease?
> 189 said yes, 2 said no, 2 were uncertain; once more 98 percent affirmative.

With such agreement by the top scientists connecting dietary cholesterol with the blood level of cholesterol and heart disease, I fail to find room for controversy.

But What About HDL Cholesterol—Isn't It More Important Than the Total Level?

Actually, no. HDL levels are not more important than total cholesterol levels, but they certainly are important.

Cholesterol is a small molecule that travels in the blood attached to larger complexes of fat and protein. There are three major carriers of cholesterol: a very light, almost-all-fat carrier called VLDL (very-low-density lipoprotein); a light carrier, also mostly fat, called LDL (low-density lipoprotein and by far the most dangerous fraction); and a heavier carrier made up of protein and fat called HDL (high-density lipoprotein, by far the more desirable fraction). Therefore, in order to get the total cholesterol level one needs to add up the various amounts of cholesterol that are carried in these three fractions.

The HDL cholesterol are the good guys. This fraction of cholesterol seems to mobilize cholesterol out of the arteries and take it to the liver, where it is converted into bile and excreted. People with very high levels of HDL cholesterol are less prone to have heart attacks. The LDL cholesterol is the major culprit. This is the fraction of cholesterol that deposits into the wall of the artery and brings on atherosclerosis and its associated misery. Therefore, elevated levels of LDL cholesterol are exceedingly dangerous.

Take for example two men: Each has a total cholesterol level of 240, but one man has an LDL cholesterol of approximately 180 with an HDL cholesterol of approximately 40. The other man has an LDL cholesterol of approximately 160, with an HDL cholesterol fraction of 60. They each have cholesterol levels of 240, yet the first gentleman has a significantly higher risk of having a heart attack than does the second gentleman because a lower percentage of his cholesterol is carried in the safe HDL fraction.

The best way to correlate the two is by a ratio. If the total cholesterol level is divided by the HDL cholesterol, then that number has a predictive value of risk. For instance, a total cholesterol level of 240 with an HDL cholesterol of 40 gives a ratio of 6.0. This is about the average risk. The gentleman with a total cholesterol level of 240 and an HDL of 60 gives a ratio of 4.0 which is measurably lower.

These ratios of risk using the HDL and total cholesterol levels are somewhat helpful within the American population that has very high levels. However, in other populations that have a total cholesterol level around 140 to 160, the ratios are irrelevant because the bad cholesterol, the LDL fraction, is so low as rarely to promote atherosclerosis.

The question now is, What dietary or other measures exist to lower the LDL fraction (which are the bad guys) and elevate the

HDL fraction (which are the good guys)? As early as 1954 Dr. Ancel Keys noted that the Japanese on their traditional low-fat diet had HDL cholesterol levels of 40.3 with a very low LDL fraction of 120.3 for a total cholesterol level ranging from 150 to 170. However, when the Japanese migrated to America and began eating the American diet, the HDL cholesterol dropped to 35.2 and the LDL shot up to 212 for a total cholesterol level in excess of 250.

It is generally recognized that vegetarians have much lower LDL cholesterol (the bad guys) and far more favorable ratios between total cholesterol level and HDL. It has also been shown that exercise has a tendency to elevate the HDL fraction of cholesterol as do certain vitamins and minerals including niacin and in some studies vitamin C. What is also crystal clear is that a diet high in saturated fat and cholesterol dramatically elevates the LDL or dangerous fraction.

The Final Piece of the Puzzle

Surely the most important study on blood cholesterol level and heart disease was the Lipid Research Clinic's coronary primary prevention trial; it was completed and published in January 1984 (*JAMA*, 251: 351–374, 1984). In order to understand the significance of this study, let's set the stage.

We have known since the turn of the century that cholesterol and fat added to the diet of rabbits, guinea pigs, or monkeys (very close to human beings) would without question cause the very blockages in the arteries that are seen in humans who suffer from heart disease. In addition, we have known that these animals would then develop the same problems that human beings suffer, namely, heart attacks, congestive heart failure, and sudden death. Firmly established evidence has more recently indicated, as a corollary to this animal research, that the atherosclerotic blockages in these animals would reverse if the animals were given a low-fat diet that significantly lowered their blood cholesterol level.

We have also known for many years that heart disease is reserved almost exclusively for Western cultures, which consume generous amounts of fat and cholesterol in their diets. In comparison with other cultures, such as the Japanese, who eat low levels of fat and cholesterol, the high-fat, high-cholesterol consumption of the American is quite distinct. This type of American diet, as I have said over and over in this book, causes elevation of the blood cholesterol level in comparison to the Japanese and other Oriental cultures (American cholesterol average, 210 to 220; Japanese cholesterol average, 150 to 160). We have also known for some time that when the Japanese come to this country and eat our high-fat diet, their cholesterol levels immediately skyrocket to our dangerous level and they immediately have an increased risk of death from cardiovascular disease. (This risk equals ours within one generation, an amazing ten-fold increase.)

Over the last two decades we have documented clearly that the cholesterol levels in the blood are highly predictive of impending heart attacks—those with cholesterol levels of 260 or higher are far more likely to have heart attacks than those with cholesterol levels of 210 or lower. There is a clearly established risk of heart attack that increases with each increase in the blood cholesterol level.

The sum total of this evidence is so strong that for years the American Heart Association and other physicians have strongly advised us to reduce the fat and cholesterol in our diet as a preventive measure against heart disease.

Nonetheless, there were still detractors to these recommendations for dietary changes. The final piece of the puzzle was absent; it had never been shown that if one were to lower the blood cholesterol level of a group known to be a high risk of having a heart attack, their risk would be reduced. The National Institute of Health undertook to answer that very question. They recruited 3,806 men with no history of heart disease but who were known to be high-risk candidates for heart attack and whose cholesterol levels were 265 or higher. I might point out here—again—that 265 is still considered normal by many physicians and laboratories even though it is known to carry a very high risk of heart death. The researchers contemplated doing a study of dietary changes that would lower the cholesterol level but ruled against this method for the following reasons.

First, the study was designed to last 7 years (it lasted 7.4 years) and the researchers knew that it would be difficult for the experimental group to stick to a low-fat diet—even though it was healthy—for that long period of time in order to lower their cholesterol levels enough to make a difference. Also, the researchers wanted to have the study double-blinded—that is, they did not want either the volunteers or the researchers themselves to know which group were receiving the cholesterol-lowering therapy. Obviously it would be easy for volunteers and researchers to figure who was on the low-cholesterol diet.

For these reasons the researchers chose a drug called Questran that can be used to lower the cholesterol in the blood. It has a binding effect on cholesterol in the intestinal tract, increasing its excretion and thereby lowering the blood levels. The 3,806 volunteers were divided into two groups, half receiving Questran, the other half receiving a placebo. Both groups were put on a moderate cholesterol-lowering diet.

At the end of the study, the results were truly astounding! Those taking the Questran had a definite reduction in cholesterol levels in comparison to the control—8.5 percent reduction. This reduction translated into a reduced death rate of 19 percent, a greater than two-to-one ratio. Those taking the cholesterol-lowering agent also had significantly less angina (20 percent), a reduced incidence of positive stress test (25 percent), and a significant reduction in ultimate bypass surgery (21 percent) in comparison to the control. In short, every manifestation of heart disease was reduced by lowering the blood cholesterol level with Questran.

The researchers were quick to point out that even though the study used a cholesterol-lowering drug, these same results would be expected if the cholesterol level were lowered by diet. They also extrapolated that the significant reduction of death achieved by lowering the blood cholesterol level would also be expected in patients with much lower cholesterol levels—in the 200 to 250 range.

The final piece of the puzzle was found and it fit perfectly—more perfectly than anyone had imagined!

Egg Yolks and Lecithin

Isn't it true that egg yolks contain lecithin, which protects you from cholesterol?

There is considerable confusion about lecithin which itself is a fat, phospholipid. In the body, cholesterol can attach to a lecithin molecule and in this regard lecithin acts like a detergent, at least theoretically, keeping cholesterol mobilized, protecting against deposits of cholesterol on the artery wall. However, studies with lecithin supplements have been disappointing. Dr. H. F. ter Welle fed 2 to 4 grams of soya lecithin to twelve patients with high cholesterol levels and found no change. In fact, the researchers felt that the lecithin as the dietary supplement was not even absorbed.

The true role of lecithin is yet to be defined, but one thing is certain—for lecithin to have any effect it must be an unsaturated lecithin from a vegetable source such as soya lecithin. Cholesterol is attached to a lecithin molecule at the unsaturated bond between two carbon atoms. If the lecithin is animal-derived, it is already saturated at this site and cannot bond with a cholesterol molecule, and even theoretically has no effect.

Almost all the lecithin in an egg yolk is saturated (as are most fats from animal origin). Therefore, even if soya lecithin or other vegetable lecithins are found to be beneficial or protective against heart disease, egg yolk lecithin cannot be so because it is a saturated, animal-derived fat. In fact, studies have shown that this animal-derived lecithin, which is saturated, actually promotes atherosclerosis, and rather than being protective has even been demonstrated to elevate the cholesterol level in the blood as a result of egg yolk consumption.

10

Where Will I Get My Protein?

The most common question concerning this mostly vegetarian program is, Where will I get my protein? Almost from birth we are taught that substantial amounts of animal protein are essential to meet protein requirements, and without these animal protein foods one can expect a health disaster. The mere suggestion of eliminating meat, eggs, and dairy products usually causes panic. Ironically, it is these very animal protein foods that predictably destroy health. Yet even in those who already suffer from the high-protein American diet, there is still the fear of some dire consequences when these animal protein foods are eliminated. To dismantle these completely irrational fears, let's (1) examine the fear and (2) establish your actual protein requirements.

The Fear

If you at this time were suffering from protein deficiency, what might your problem be? Anemia? That's not a protein deficiency problem. Anemia results from blood loss, inadequate iron replacement, B_{12} or folic acid deficiency, but not from protein deficiency. Hair loss? Hair loss results from a variety of changes none of which are a specific protein deficiency. Deterioration of the body? Generally the body deterioration that occurs from starvation is just that, not an isolated protein deficiency. Secondly, excessive protein intake is not necessary to build or maintain bulky muscles. This occurs with weight lifting exercises and simply by eating enough food. There is no need for a high-protein diet. Loss of energy? This myth is particularly widespread and has led to all manner of high-protein concoctions supposedly to boost energy. Energy is required to move around, and to do so, your muscles burn carbohydrate and fat calories exclusively. You never, repeat never, burn protein calories for energy. Even in the throes of starvation when protein is required for energy, it is first converted into carbohydrates and then utilized. However, this occurs only during starvation or when for some reason carbohydrates are eliminated from the diet.

Generally, the possibility of actual protein deficiency occurring in the American population is very slight indeed. The fear of protein deficiency, however, perpetuates continued excessive consumption of meat, eggs, and dairy products, the foods which almost exclusively bring on heart disease, angina pectoris, high blood pressure, diabetes, stroke, and contribute to a host of other conditions including osteoporosis, obesity, and kidney failure. Let's now determine how much protein you actually need.

How Much Protein Do You Need?

You obviously need protein in your daily nutrition, and that protein is used to maintain body tissue. It is a common misconception that because the majority of your tissues are made of protein, you need to eat a lot of protein for maintenance of your body. Your body is very efficient at using and reusing the protein available to it; therefore, the actual amount for maintenance is very small.

Even during growth, the amount of protein required is much smaller than is generally imagined. We often forget that vegetable foods contain substantial amounts of body-building protein. Have you ever wondered where the protein of horses, cows, and other animals comes from if all they eat is grass? In order to bring some sense to the mythology around protein requirements, let's examine the actual protein need.

The Food and Nutrition Board of the National Academy of Science has estimated that the requirement of protein for the average adult is about fifty-five grams for women and sixty-five grams for men. They point out that a total vegetarian man takes in 128 percent of his protein requirements, while a total vegetarian woman takes in 111 percent of her protein requirements. They go on to point out that their recommendation for protein is deliberately set at twice the amount of protein demonstrated to be adequate in the adult. Therefore, the complete vegetarian man or woman is taking in well over 200 percent of his or her protein requirements. It is virtually impossible for a vegetarian who is getting enough calories and eating a diversity of vegetable foods ever to be protein-deficient.

The World Health Organization and the Food and Agriculture Organization routinely make estimates and subsequent recommendations for the daily intake of protein for an adult. The most recent protein recommendations for the adult were to ingest approximately one-half gram of protein per kilogram of body weight. Therefore, the adult weighing 150 pounds (70 kilograms) would require about 35 grams of protein per day. The complete vegetarian who eats between 2,100 and 2,600 calories of various foods would be taking in between 65 and 80 grams of protein per day, close to 200 percent more than the adequate amount. For the American consuming 100 to 120 grams per day, however, he is 300 to 400 percent over his protein needs.

The Essential Amino Acid Myth

It's commonly believed that many vegetable foods lack some of the essential amino acids. These essential amino acids are protein-building blocks that must be derived from food because the body cannot synthesize them. This myth is so strong that vegetarians take great pains to balance their vegetable foods. Actually, every vegetable food contains all of the essential amino acids, but some vegetable foods contain lower amounts of certain amino acids. In practice, however, this is not very important.

As Dr. D. M. Hegsted pointed out in 1976 in a letter to the editor of the *American Journal of Clinical Nutrition,* "The quality of dietary protein is of little or no significance unless dietary protein is of very poor quality comparable to that of white flour. This is consistent with the evidence that the adult requirements for essential amino acids are very low relative to the total nitrogen need."

To me, this myth about the need to balance vegetable foods

represents the vegetarian paranoia. Hopelessly outnumbered and constantly harassed by meat eaters, the vegetarian feels compelled to demonstrate that combining certain vegetable foods duplicates the balance of animal protein. Frances Moore Lappé in her widely read book *Diet for a Small Planet* gave detailed techniques for food combining to ensure balanced protein. In her most recent book, *Diet for a Small Planet Revisited,* she points out that balancing vegetable proteins is not necessary; one need only to eat enough diversified vegetable foods.

Most Americans don't realize that breads, cereals, potatoes, corn, oatmeal, vegetables, rice, and legumes are not only carbohydrates, but also excellent sources of protein. Here at the Institute it is a never-ending task convincing patients that a complete meal of these so-called carbohydrate foods is more than adequate in protein.

The actual requirement of the essential amino acids by an adult is surprisingly low. The World Health Organization recommends that 15 percent of the recommended 35 grams of protein for the 150-pound adult be in the form of essential amino acids. This equals 5.25 grams or the amount of essential amino acids that would be contained in about 6 ounces of nonfat milk. However, a complete complement of essential amino acids would also be supplied on an all-vegetable food diet if adequate calories were maintained.

Protein Poisoning

The real protein problem in this country is protein poisoning from ingesting too much protein. To understand the toxicity of excessive protein in the body you must know how the body handles the carbohydrates, fats, and protein that are present in any diet.

Carbohydrates and fats are made up of carbon, hydrogen, and oxygen. The basic carbohydrate is glucose, which contains six carbon atoms, twelve hydrogen atoms, and six oxygen atoms. Starches or complex carbohydrates are glucose and other sugars that are hooked together. Linoleic acid is a basic fat and contains eighteen carbon atoms, thirty-two hydrogen atoms, and two oxygen atoms. Both fats and carbohydrates are burned for energy, and their breakdown products are carbon dioxide, which is eliminated by the lungs, and water, which can be used by the body or eliminated by the kidneys. Excessive amounts of carbohydrates or fats can be stored in the body in the form of fat. This is an efficient method of storing energy against a food shortage, but since so many of us never run into a real shortage in our civilized world, we keep piling up that stored fat.

The body handles protein very differently. Proteins contain not only carbon, hydrogen, and oxygen, but also nitrogen, sulphur, and phosphorus. Proteins are never used for energy, except during severe starvation, and are needed only to replace the daily protein losses of the body. Only small amounts of protein are needed to maintain health. Since we Americans get 400 percent of protein requirements, what does the body do with the excess? It has no way to store nitrogen, sulphur, and phosphorus. So the extra protein has to be broken down into urea and uric acid and eliminated through the kidneys.

When you take in 400 percent of your protein requirements, all of your metabolic systems are stressed by the overload. The kidneys take the worst beating. Thanksgiving may be a holiday for you, but your kidneys work overtime.

The labs have a simple way to assess how well a set of kidneys is functioning. They test a sample of the person's blood and measure the amounts of circulating protein breakdown products in it. Healthy kidneys keep the BUN—blood, urea, nitrogen—and that other protein-breakdown product, creatinine—at low levels in the blood. When abused kidneys fail, the BUN and creatinine levels rise and the body is poisoned.

Excessive Protein and Kidney Failure

The kidneys are remarkable organs with a lot of reserve capacity. Generally they are able to handle the excessive protein that is a byproduct of our way of life. But when other diseases damage the kidneys the excess protein speeds up kidney failure. Diabetes and high blood pressure damage the kidneys, and people with these disorders often suffer complete kidney failure and require kidney transplants or chronic dialysis.

This disaster could be delayed or perhaps prevented altogether if these patients were started early on lower protein diets.

Dr. W. E. Mitch and his colleagues at the Brigham and Women's

Hospital in Boston studied the effects of a very-low-protein diet on twenty-four persons with moderately advanced kidney failure. There were various reasons for the kidney failure, including high blood pressure, diabetes, and chronic glomerulonephritis—a progressively advancing kidney disease. The diet included mostly vegetables and slight amounts of amino acid supplements that totaled twenty to thirty grams of protein a day. In seventeen of the twenty-four patients, this dietary regime significantly slowed the rate of deterioration. In seven of the patients the deterioration was halted completely for twenty-two months. In commenting on his results, Dr. Mitch stated that the low-protein diet "slows down the ongoing loss of kidney function that seems to be characteristic of kidney disease, regardless of the kind of kidney disease the patient started with."

In Los Angeles recently at the Ninth International Congress of Nephrology, Dr. Carmelo Giordano of the University of Naples, Italy, pointed out that "up until a few years ago, dietary management of chronic renal failure was confined to those patients having little renal function—perhaps 10 percent—left. The new concept is to recommend dietary management not only for patients waiting to enter dialysis but for the estimated 2 million Americans who have created a serum creatinine of two milligrams-DL (or higher)." A two-milligram creatinine is indicative of very slight kidney dysfunction and is generally ignored in terms of recommendations of dietary management by most physicians. It is at this stage of kidney dysfunction that a low-protein diet would likely have its most beneficial effect, perhaps stopping the dysfunction completely and eliminating the enormously debilitating process of dialysis or kidney transplant that is necessary with complete kidney failure.

Protein and Calcium Loss

Excessive protein-breakdown products create an acid condition in the blood, and the body mobilizes calcium from bone to neutralize the acid. When the breakdown products are eliminated by the kidneys the mobilized calcium is eliminated also. Over a lifetime a high-protein diet steals enough calcium to weaken bones; this is the condition called osteoporosis, and it, sadly, is the reason that old bones break so easily.

Dr. Richard B. Mazess, of the Bone, Mineral Laboratory at the

University of Wisconsin, studied a group of 217 Alaskan Eskimos living on a high-protein diet of fish, marine mammals, and caribou. These folk consumed up to three times the amount of protein as average Americans. By the age of forty, this excessive protein intake had caused enough calcium loss to reduce their bone density by 10 to 15 percent compared to those in the same area on a lower protein

Dr. Ruth Walker, of the Department of Nutritional Sciences, University of Wisconsin, measured calcium loss in nine healthy young men who were ingesting three different levels of protein—47 grams a day, 95 grams a day, and 145 grams a day. All were receiving adequate calcium—the recommended daily allowance of 800 mg daily. On the lower protein intakes they were in positive calcium balance, retaining 12 mg on the lowest protein intake and 1 mg on the middle protein intake. Of their 800 daily mg of calcium, they were storing some in their bones. But the men on the high 145-gram protein diet were losing more calcium daily than they were taking in—85 mg more. The excessive protein was stealing that much from their bones, after using all of the 800-mg intake. At that rate, in forty years they would have lost 75 percent of the calcium in their skeletons.

Dr. Nancy Johnson, also of the Department of Nutritional Sciences at the University of Wisconsin, studied six normal men each taking 1,400 mg of calcium daily. This is a high calcium intake, 75 percent higher than the RDA level of 800 mg. Initially these men were given a diet containing 47 grams of protein. On this diet they were in positive calcium balance, retaining 10 mg of calcium each day. When they were shifted to a diet of 147 grams of protein, on the same amount of calcium intake, they went into negative calcium balance, losing 85 mg of calcium a day from bone.

It is clear from all these studies that calcium metabolism is more a function of protein intake than of calcium intake. This means that if you are on a high-protein diet you could be losing calcium from your bones, regardless of how much calcium you ingest.

Vegetarians Have Stronger Bones

Of all the nutritional myths, the belief that milk and meat are needed to build strong bones and teeth is likely the most inaccurate. Exactly the opposite may be the case; milk and meat in large quantities can actually cause weak bones and lost teeth. As early as 1920 it was shown that vegetarians have stronger bones than meat eaters. Because of their lower protein intake, vegetarians stay in positive calcium balance, continually adding calcium to their bones. If meat or other high-protein foods are added to the vegetarian diet, there is an immediate increase in calcium loss in the urine. The first step to building strong bones and teeth would be to reduce milk and meat, because of their high protein content.

Testimony to this fact is obvious. We all know that elderly Americans have very weak bones. Osteoporosis, the weakening of bones, is epidemic in American culture. As a result, fractures of the hip are common in the elderly, the spine collapses with age, teeth fall out, and many of our elderly shuffle around the last years of their life crippled by a deteriorating skeleton. The irony is that these individuals have been drinking milk and eating meat all of their lives!

Am I suggesting that your six-year-old stop drinking milk?

Yes, I am. The net effect of a large amount of milk even in children is more likely to be damaging than healthy. Milk from cows is poorly tolerated by many youngsters as they lack the enzyme necessary to break down the milk sugar called lactose. Secondly, cow's milk seems to be a major cause of allergic problems that lead to colic in infants, nasal congestion and ear infections in children, as well as a variety of skin disorders. These problems now are thought to continue into childhood and adolescence, and in many they disappear with elimination of milk. Aside from these complications, we must remember the role that the saturated fat in milk plays in developing atherosclerotic heart disease. Whole milk is 55 percent fat and surely elevates the blood cholesterol level of even youngsters who consume large amounts of it. After children begin eating solid food, they would be much healthier if they received their nutritional requirements of calcium and protein from nondairy sources. As we shall see, green vegetables are excellent sources of calcium.

Don't infants need milk?

Of course—mother's milk. We seem to forget that the human breast in addition to its ornamental attributes makes milk, the ideal food for human infants. Generally, infancy is the first six to eight months of life, during which time the infant doubles his weight, going from seven pounds to about fourteen pounds. No question that the ideal food, and the only food necessary, is mother's milk during this period. It provides all the nutrients necessary for this phenomenal growth phase. Imagine as an adult doubling your weight in six months!

During these six months of rapid growth the infant's protein needs are substantial, almost 400 percent that of an adult based upon body weight. However, all of this protein is provided by mother's milk which, would you believe, is a very-low-protein food, only 6 percent caloric protein. This is one of the lowest protein foods generally consumed by human beings. Cow's milk on the other hand is 22 percent caloric protein, containing 300 percent the amount of protein in mother's milk. If undiluted cow's milk were the only food for the human infant, the result would likely be fatal. Cow's milk is the ideal food for a newborn calf, and in case you haven't noticed, humans and cows are quite different.

The main point of this discussion is that even from infancy, when the protein needs of human beings are the highest, the human system is designed generally for low-protein foods. When this rapid-growth phase levels off and the protein requirements drop, it is sheer insanity to assume that foods containing three to five times the protein concentration of mother's milk are then necessary.

If the facts and figures of milk consumption are not enough to convince you that milk is inappropriate in the adult diet, ask yourself this question: What other mammal continues to drink milk after it is weaned? Only man. And man doesn't even drink his own milk but robs it from a cow. If milk were such good food for the adult mammal then we would see adult cows suckling each other.

If no milk, where would I get my calcium?

It may not matter how much calcium is in your diet. For example, cultures who consume a much lower amount of calcium seem to have stronger bones and teeth than Americans who consume substantially higher amounts of calcium. Western man who drinks a lot of milk takes in 800 to 1,000 mg of calcium a day, half of it coming from milk. The Bantu Africans who drink no milk at all take in only 175 to 475 mg of calcium daily. Yet comparative studies show that the Bantu have healthier teeth and stronger, denser bones than Western Americans.

Also, the expert committee from the World Health Organization and Food and Agriculture Organization stated in 1962 that "... no clear cut disease due to calcium deficiency has ever been described in the human male."

Be that as it may, most Americans are still brainwashed by the dairy industry, thinking that milk is the only source of calcium in the diet. All things considered, a better source of calcium are the leafy green vegetables. In fact, they have more calcium per calorie than milk. Whole milk contains 1.8 mg of calcium per calorie while parsley contains 4.6 mg of calcium per calorie. Spinach contains 3.6 mg of calcium per calorie and lowly romaine lettuce contains 3.6 mg of calcium per calorie. Watercress is particularly high in calcium, containing 7.9 mg per calorie. All green vegetables are excellent sources of calcium.

When calcium is derived from vegetable sources, the amount of phosphorus present is reduced. Many researchers point out that the high phosphorus intake of a meat diet increases the calcium deficiency and weakens the bones. Meat is very high in phosphorus which makes it a poor source for calcium. When the calcium/phosphorus ratio is measured, green vegetables are far superior as a source of calcium without phosphorus. For instance, in meat the calcium/phosphorus ratio is 1.3 to 1, while green vegetables have the far superior calcium/phosphorus ratio of 3.6 to 1.

It seems to be clear from the research relating protein and calcium metabolism that protein is far more important in determining calcium balance than is the actual amount of calcium in the diet. Rather than encouraging people to consume dairy products, we should educate them to reduce their protein intake. I would like now to summarize the following important points about protein nutrition:

1. The average American consumes 100 to 120 grams of protein daily, mostly from animal sources.
2. Protein requirements for humans are satisfied with 35 to 50 grams of protein per day. All of the protein requirements, including the essential amino acids, are easily satisfied by a diversified vegetable food diet that supplies adequate calories.
3. The body cannot store extra protein. This protein must be broken down into urea and other protein breakdown products and excreted in the urine.
4. Excessive protein puts a constant stress on the kidney and can accelerate kidney disease and kidney failure that are a complication of diabetes, high blood pressure, and other diseases.

5. The protein breakdown products create an acid condition in the blood which leaches calcium out of the bone, causing excessive calcium loss. This relationship makes the protein intake more important to calcium metabolism and calcium balance than is calcium intake in human cultures.

6. Because high-protein diets cause calcium loss, the American population suffers from an epidemic of osteoporosis and poor dental health. Vegetarians have long been known to have stronger bones and teeth than meat eaters.

7. Every major killer disease of Americans—heart disease, cancer, high blood pressure, diabetes—is increased by excessive amounts of meat and animal protein, and decreased when animal protein foods are replaced with vegetable foods.

PART II

Reversing the Damage

11

The Institute Program

Now that the causes of heart disease are clearly understood, we come to the solution. The purpose of this book is to show that nutrition, exercise, and appropriate medications are not alternatives to the high-technology approach to heart disease, but are absolutely essential for successful management. Our modern hospitals and highly skilled cardiologists create the belief that nutrition may be helpful, but *real* medicine involves some kind of fancy but dangerous tests and an expensive, even more dangerous, operation. That belief is not only inaccurate, but dangerous and counterproductive.

Heart disease and atherosclerosis are diffuse, progressive problems. A program of diet, exercise, and complete risk-factor control is the only approach that systematically attacks the cause of this problem. To ignore this is just plain stupid in the light of current research and scientific studies.

As Dr. Antonio M. Gotto, president of the American Heart Association, stated in *Cardiovascular News* (April 1984), "... diet remains the first form of treatment whether patients with heart disease have high levels of [blood] cholesterol or borderline cases of 240 mgs."

What is needed is a dramatic shift of priorities. For the majority of patients who have symptoms of cardiovascular disease or who have just had a heart attack, the angiogram or bypass surgery should not be considered until they have had vigorous treatment with diet, exercise, and appropriate medications. Here at the Institute this shift in priorities is evident in every aspect of treatment: the patient is not confined in a hospital environment, and the role of the physician is more that of an educator than a skilled purveyor of fancy tests.

The Institute Program

An illness is not an abstraction—it happens to a human being. In the age of high-tech medicine many doctors get by without considering the humanity of their "cases." This is particularly unfortunate in dealing with heart disease and related illnesses, because the only cure possible is something the patient must do for himself or herself. The doctor is essentially a guide, a monitor, and most importantly, a teacher. I remind you that the word "doctor" *means* one who teaches. "Curing" people with sick arteries is not done by running some tests, doing some fancy plumbing work, or simply handing the patient a prescription to be filled at the pharmacy. The doctor has to talk, to answer questions, to take a very personal interest in getting the patient to change his unhealthy habits. That means watching the patient learn the ropes, understand the principles of a complete approach, and helping him build enthusiasm for it.

When I started the Institute in 1979, I wanted a comfortable place where patients could learn the basics of nutrition in a group experience, where education was emphasized, where the patients could experience the food themselves and realize short-term benefits, which would motivate them to continue the program at home. My intention was to take patients with cardiovascular disease, diabetes, and high blood pressure, turn them in the right direction with dietary and life-style changes, and send them back to their own physician for continued care. I certainly do not envision this Institute as a substitute for a hospital or diagnostic center. Without question, the hospital is the best place to be if and when a heart attack hits, and it also has the latest technology available for sophisticated diagnostic procedures. I wanted the Institute to fill the void that this technical approach to the treatment of heart disease has created—so that patients with this disease can get the education and motivation necessary to change their life-style successfully.

With over 58 million people suffering from heart or blood vessel diseases, and literally thousands of hospitals displaying the latest technology in the management of the crises that develop, the almost total absence of institutions designed to change patients' eating habits is astounding. As Dr. William Castelli, director of the Framingham heart studies, has pointed out, we need new and creative methods for teaching diet and exercise therapy, for "bringing diet therapy back into the mainstream of medicine."

A Typical Day at the Institute

It starts early—8:00 A.M. for "vitals." Patients weigh in, have their blood pressure and pulse recorded, and give a history of the day before—how far each walked, the pulse rate attained during exercise, and a rundown of any symptoms experienced. These daily reports help us to evaluate progress and alter medication dosage.

8:30 A.M. Breakfast, which could be almond oatmeal, pancakes, French toast (egg whites only), or cold cereal with the ever present oatmeal muffins, fresh fruit, and vitamin supplements.

9:15 A.M. to 10:00 A.M. Three times weekly each patient is individually evaluated. Medications are often changed; insulin is almost always reduced in a gradual manner as are numerous heart and blood pressure drugs. This is done only with close monitoring of the blood sugar and blood pressure. Also, the patient's individual laboratory tests are discussed as are all aspects of each particular case. We believe that patient education and open discussion about all aspects of the treatment are essential to the practice of medicine.

10:00 A.M. to 10:45 A.M. Scheduled exercise. Most patients exercise throughout the day but each morning at 10:00 the group exercises together and they are monitored by the staff. During this time we can determine if each patient is taking the pulse accurately, is exercising at an appropriate level, and if he or she should decrease or increase activity. Symptoms are also checked "in the field" which gives the staff a good sense of how each patient is doing.

Noon. Lunch. It could be Mexican burritos, Chinese vegetables with rice, corn chowder with salad and bread, nonfat pizza, or a host of other pleasing and healthy dishes.

1:30 P.M. to 2:30 P.M. Seminar. Each day a specific subject is discussed, such as heart disease, the bypass operation, diabetes, the reversal of atherosclerosis, the cholesterol controversy, etc. It is during these seminar sessions that patients begin to understand their problem as well as the role the diet and exercise program plays in their improvement. These seminars inform and motivate patients to follow the program at home. Some of the session deals with food preparation for the family so that, in addition to printed recipes and menus, patients clearly understand the mechanics of following this program at home. These sessions are the backbone of this program. Each session has also been recorded on tape and every patient is given the complete series. This provides re-enforcement and program recall after they return home. Because friends of former patients have heard these tapes and have requested copies from the Institute, these tapes are now available to anyone wishing to have a personal copy of the series.

4:00 P.M. Relaxation time. Patients gather to undergo a special relaxation session. Each lies on a foam rubber mat and is guided in progressive relaxation. The purpose is to train patients in relaxation techniques to help overcome stress and to guide them in "health visualization," which is actually visualizing oneself as healthy, active, thin, without pain or medication. We realize that stress plays a role in disease and these relaxation visualization sessions are useful in controlling the contribution stress adds to disease. Patients enjoy this peaceful interlude at the end of the day.

5:30 P.M. Dinner. This is a time to enjoy the end of a day of accomplishment. Dinner is served in the main dining room. The delicious healthful meal is enjoyed with good fellowship and leisurely conversation.

Oxygen: At various times all patients breathe oxygen from an oxygen tank. As mentioned before, breathing oxygen helps to reverse atherosclerosis. Some patients ride a stationary bicycle while breathing oxygen, others read and relax. Most report that it makes them feel better.

Many patients, particularly diabetic patients, have such poor circulation in their legs that open ulcers develop. This often leads to amputation. To heal the ulcers and avoid this complication, patients spend at least one hour daily with their legs in a pressurized oxygen tank. The tank fills with 100 percent oxygen under pressure and releases the pressure every fifteen seconds. The oxygen which is humidified is forced by the pressure into the open ulcer, which rapidly begins to heal. Sometimes ulcers that have been getting worse for months will heal in a matter of weeks.

Obviously, the days are full and active. For the first time, patients spend the whole day doing things to improve their health. Many accomplished and disciplined people, expert in their field, limp into the Institute riddled with heart disease, diabetes, high blood pressure, and other serious problems. For many, this is their first experience in improving their health and concentrating on the needs of their body. They quickly understand that their body is a wonderful, finely tuned miracle that must be cared for. They are eager to learn how to reverse the diseases which have taken their toll.

Observations of the Doctor

After observing about 2,000 patients start and complete this program, I have seen some general changes that occur in patients while in the Institute:

1. *First several days:* Almost everyone is a little skeptical about the Institute because it doesn't feel like a hospital or fit the general picture. However, most are convinced that this approach makes a lot of sense and have decided before their arrival to give it a try. There is a lot of testing in the first few days—complete physical examination, blood test, exercise test, etc. Patients meet the other members of the group and often talk about why they came and what they hope to get out of the program. They begin to make friends rapidly. Everyone is in the same boat, going in the same direction, with the same goal—to regain their health.

2. *End of first week:* The mood is considerably lighter. Information in the seminars convinces patients of the benefits of a more active life-style. For a few, improvements have already begun—a little less angina, more physical endurance, less insulin, etc. Friendships are becoming stronger and a group spirit begins to form. Even though each comes from a different walk of life and will return to such, they're all learning the same thing: how to alter their life-style in key areas to regain and maintain their health. This is fertile ground for camaraderie.

3. *Start of the second week:* The second week is different from the first. The routine of activities, exercise, oxygen, and relaxation has been established and patients now concentrate on improvements. During this last week many medications and symptoms are gone. Patients who had never walked a mile, and considered it im-

possible, are walking two to three miles without difficulty. An interim blood test generally shows improvement which would include a much lower cholesterol level and lower blood sugar. Blood pressures are down and most have lost some excess weight. Seminars continue to give more information and serve to reinforce each patient's commitment to the program. Most are already planning how to handle the business lunch, shopping, and when and how they will do their exercise. For the most part, the patients are continually surprised at how pleasant the food can be. They have experienced a wide variety of food, many of which they had considered taboo: pancakes, waffles, spaghetti, potatoes, even potatoes baked in strips that taste like French fries.

4. *End of the program:* As patients complete this program, there is a sense of enthusiasm and a marked change in attitude.

First, fear, which often immobilizes the heart patient, is replaced with a resolve to lick the problem. Heart patients are not deluded about the seriousness of their problem. Quite the contrary. They understand even more clearly how dangerous it is. However, they now have a plan of action: it's one thing to be continually afraid, quite another to be appropriately concerned with a specific plan that has already started to work. Second, the life-style changes are no longer viewed as arduous or impossible. Actually, most view the program as an opportunity, even a challenge, to overcome their problems. There is an increase in the respect one has for his body and ultimately even for himself. The poisonous high-fat foods so common in our culture are avoided for the simple reason: Why would anyone do that to himself. Health now becomes a game and a high priority. The diet, exercise, and vitamin programs become the tools in winning. Third, and most important, patients are no longer passive consumers of drugs, constantly in the dark about their problems. They are now active partners in their health care. They are trained in taking their blood pressure and pulse, and they understand the importance of certain laboratory values such as the cholesterol level, triglyceride level, and blood sugar. They realize the integral role nutrition will play in their recovery, and they are determined to receive the benefits of exercise.

When these patients return to the care of their local physician, they are "model patients" who really want to get better. This change in attitude occasionally creates friction, and some physicians are upset by this more aggressive resolve to improve; but most physicians welcome the changes: "John, I've been trying to get you to do this for years."

In the final analysis, these changes in attitude are essential for any long-term success. The structured environment, regulated activities, and the group interaction here at the Institute are designed to affect these important attitude changes. Almost all patients state that they could never have made the necessary changes without the structured input and group interaction.

12

The Nutrition Program

At first glance this program may look impossible. The diet looks Spartan and you can't imagine ever liking to eat this way. This first reaction is normal when starting any change in dietary patterns. However, as you learn more and become more experienced while your body adjusts to the changes, it becomes easier until finally you not only like the food, but you've given up the cravings for the unhealthy foods you left behind.

I do not underestimate the effort that is required in getting started and adjusting to this dietary regimen. It's not easy. If it were, it would be of precious little benefit to you or anyone else. The entire thrust of this book is a clarion call to change our nutritional habits that are responsible for making people ill. Changing nutritional habits is more difficult than changing any other form of habitual behavior.

There are two philosophies on how to approach dietary change. One is for individuals to ease into a dietary change: to cut meat consumption from five nights a week to twice a week, to reduce consumption of cheese to once a week, and to cut down to two eggs a week, and to go from there gradually reducing the offending foods.

Another philosophy is to immerse the patient in the optimum dietary program designed to give the maximum benefit. This means making no compromises at the beginning and setting up a detailed, structured program for the patient to follow. I personally believe this latter approach is more successful for two reasons.

First, how many alcoholics do you know who control their habit by drinking moderately, or how many smokers are able simply to cut down the number of cigarettes? Obviously the avenue for success in these two addictions is simply to stop. Many of our food habits are the same and require the same degree of discipline, particularly at first.

For many of my patients, the disease has already reached such a level of seriousness that one can no longer take it lightly. The diet program that we use at the Institute and that is offered in this book is designed for maximum benefit in the shortest amount of time. As such, it is very powerful in lowering the cholesterol level and producing the other benefits outlined. For instance, Dr. Dean Ornish used a diet almost identical to the one described in this book, along with mild stress-reduction techniques, in heart patients over a twenty-four-day study. He found that in only twenty-four days there was a 20.5-percent reduction in plasma cholesterol level, a 91-percent reduction in frequency of angina attacks, 44-percent increase in duration of exercise, and a 55-percent increase in total work performed by the heart muscle. The patients enrolled in this study were already receiving the current medical management of this disease with various medications.

The rapidity with which beneficial and significant changes occur is quite astounding to many patients who take this type of dietary regimen. With this rapid improvement, patients who are frightened and debilitated by cardiovascular disease then become enthusiastic and motivated about strict adherence to the regimen.

In either case there is general negativity and a feeling of hopelessness when viewing the task at hand. This food, at least on paper, appears strange and unappetizing. Most of this is psychological in that you have never considered utilizing these foods as a major source of your calories or as the major entrée to a meal. However, once you get into it you realize that beans, mushrooms, and other substitutes for meat work surprisingly well. Moreover, with time you will learn to even enjoy these foods. In a very real sense, initial negativity stems more from a lack of experience than from the foods themselves.

With time, this new program will become familiar and your taste buds and preferences will have changed. You will actually be enjoying and preferring these foods and this life-style. Being human, you will get off track on occasion and when you do, it will only remind you of how far you have come, how much you have changed. For instance, after several weeks on this dietary regimen, the regular salted popcorn served in the movie houses will just about knock your head off. You will wonder how you ever tolerated such a large amount of salt in the past. You will know you have arrived when this "diet" is not a "diet," but simply the way you eat.

Of the thousands of patients who have completed this program at the Institute, without exception those who enjoy the most success and get the most pleasure out of their new regimen are those who do not look upon this regimen as a deprivation, but rather as an opportunity to improve their health and enhance their lives. Their continuing good health becomes a hobby—an avocation, and a labor of love. In some cases people will begin to treat themselves almost as well as they treat their automobiles.

Calculating Caloric Fat Percentage

In order to reduce your fat intake consistently you must first know how to calculate the percentage of fat calories in food. Most food labels contain the calories in a serving and also list the grams of carbohydrates, fat, and protein. In order to calculate the percentage of calories provided by fat, you must first convert the weight of fat in grams to calories of fat. The conversion factor is 9, meaning that 1 gram of fat contains 9 calories.

Generally, fat is the only nutrient you will need to monitor constantly as far as percentage is concerned. However, you should know how to calculate the percentage of calories that come from carbohydrates and proteins as well. Both carbohydrates and proteins have the same conversion factor of 4, meaning that there are 4 calories in each gram of carbohydrate and protein.

Obviously fat has much more caloric density than either carbohydrates or protein. One gram of fat contains 225 percent more calories than a gram of either carbohydrate or protein. This is the major reason Americans are so fat as a nation. By generously using butter or sour cream on a very healthy, low-calorie baked potato (only 80 calories) we convert it into a 350-calorie disaster.

The best way to learn how to calculate percentage of fat calories in food is simply to do it several times. Here are three examples taken from nutrition labels on commonly eaten foods which will show you how.

Example 1—Miracle Whip Salad Dressing.

Total calories per serving—70
Fat per tablespoon—7 grams
Therefore, 7 grams of fat per serving contains 9 calories per gram which equals (9 × 7) 63 calories of fat. That means that 63 of the 70 calories are fat calories.

To find the percentage of fat, divide the fat calories by the total calories in the serving, or rather 63 divided by 70 equals .9 or 90 percent.

The salad dressing is 90 percent fat.

Example 2—Campbell's Cream of Mushroom Soup.

Total calories per serving—120
Fat per serving—8 grams

Therefore, 8 grams of fat per serving times 9 calories per gram equals 72 calories of fat. That means that 72 of the 120 calories are fat calories. To find the overall percentage, divide 72 fat calories by 120 total calories which equals .60 or 60 percent.

The soup is 60 percent fat. Who said canned soup was good food?

Example 3—Spoon-size Shredded Wheat by Nabisco.

Total calories per serving—110
Fat per serving—1 gram

One gram of fat per serving times 9 calories per gram equals 9 calories of fat. That means that 9 of the 110 calories are fat calories. To find the overall percentage divide the fat calories by the total calories in the serving; 9 divided by 110 equals .082 or 8.2 percent. This cereal is only 8.2 percent fat calories. The goal of this program is for your general nutrition to contain no more than 15 percent fat calories. Therefore the salad dressing and the soup should be avoided while you can consume the shredded wheat freely.

Eating Out

This program in no way means that you have to give up dining in restaurants and using a restaurant outing as a focus of a social event. It is even possible to eat in restaurants and follow this program to a tee and still enjoy yourself. Here are some tips that will make it easier:

1. Order precisely what you want and be sure that the waiter understands you. This is the time to be polite but very specific, and almost all waiters will respect this attitude.
2. Generally, the better restaurants are more amenable to your requests and desires than are the lower-priced ones. In fact the lower you go on the price scale and the more convenience foods are served, the less likely you are to be able to get low-fat, healthy food. For that matter, you can simply eliminate all of the fast-food outlets specializing in hamburgers, fries, and fried chicken.
3. Even in the so-called steak houses you will generally find a salad bar and the menu will list some form of vegetable and a baked potato hopefully. For the purist, a baked potato, bread, and a salad bar will suffice very nicely. I have feasted this way too many times to count and therefore know it can be done.
4. Also, in most restaurants white fish is generally available and you can have it boiled, baked, or poached. Be sure to request that no fats, butter, or other oils are added to its preparation. You will find these tips to be very helpful and will often cut your restaurant bill. Once I was dining in an expensive Mexican restaurant with a lady friend of a similar dietary persuasion and we ordered from the side dish section only. Our meal consisted of Mexican rice, salad, bread, and an order of beans which were prepared without lard. The entrées in this particular restaurant started at about $7; therefore for two people to dine the bill would have been approximately $15–$20. The sum total of the bill for the both of us ordering from the side dishes only came to $4.75. I was somewhat embarrassed and left a $4 tip.

Traveling

Traveling represents a challenge at first. Some have told me that traveling and eating a low-fat diet is an absolute impossibility. Others report that traveling and eating a low-fat diet is quite easy. The difference is not in the travel but in the individuals. Since I do a considerable amount of traveling myself, I know that you can travel and continue to eat low-fat food.

Traveling is only slightly more difficult than eating out in your own town. Here are some tricks you can put to use:

*All major airlines, if given twenty-four hours notice, will provide you with special meals while in flight. While the "vegetarian" or the "low-salt, low-cholesterol" item will often suffice, I usually order a fresh fruit plate just to be safe. Second, you can always take on board with you apples, raw vegetables, and a few raw nuts, and skip the airline meals altogether. When I do this I experience a sense of independence and enjoy a better meal than the food usually dished out on airlines.

*When traveling by car your best source of snack food in an emergency is your standard supermarket. Here you can get bread, fresh fruit, raw vegetables, nonfat yogurt, and other items that can be munched in the car, or even serve as a meal or two. And, for the traveler the general rules on restaurant eating apply and are equally feasible.

Eating at Home

The bulk of the material that follows is the general guidelines for converting to low-fat nutrition at home. This information should only serve as a guideline to help you initiate the principles. There is no doubt that by following these guidelines you will be able to develop your own recipes, favorite dishes, tricks, and short cuts. But again, some simple hints often can save a lot of frustration.

If you are a cook and are familiar with food preparation you will have no problem once you get the knack of it. As in anything else, you will have successes and failures as you go along, and will develop your own short cuts and favorite recipes. If you are an experienced cook this approach will initially seem foreign but you will quickly adapt to it and even improve upon the suggested recipes in this book.

If you are an inexperienced cook then food preparation of any style is going to be difficult for you and it will take you longer to adjust to this program. However, the meals recommended in this book are no more difficult to prepare than those in any other cookbook, but I would strongly suggest that you get help in the basics before attempting the specifics of this program. The following suggestions should make home eating easier:

*Do not throw away any cookbook. Almost any recipe except those using substantial amounts of meat can be adapted to your new program. You can use some of the substitutions contained in this book for any unacceptable items or leave them out altogether.

*Prepare foods in large quantities. A lot of the soups, stews, chili, and bean dishes can be prepared in quantity and then frozen. It might even be more convenient to freeze these foods in packets of individual servings where they can be removed and prepared immediately. It is best to keep several types of frozen food available.

13

Vitamins and Minerals—the Controversy

Vitamin and mineral supplements are an integral part of the Institute's approach. However, their importance should not be overestimated; the majority of benefits come from the diet change and exercise regime. We live in a pill-pushing society, and this chapter should not create the illusion that food supplements will protect you from a high-fat, fiberless diet. Supplements are just that—a supplement to the diet and exercise program; they're not the healing factors.

There's controversy on the use of food supplements. On the one hand a strong voice is raised against using any food supplements except when there is a specific deficiency such as scurvy (vitamin C deficiency), rickets (vitamin D deficiency), or pernicious anemia (vitamin B_{12} deficiency, brought on by inability to absorb B_{12}), to mention a few. In the absence of these deficiency conditions it is assumed that the American diet (even with its dangerous excess of fat calories and cholesterol) supplies the optimum amount of the known vitamins and minerals. As stated by Dr. Victor Herbert of the Department of Medicine, Upstate University of New York, "There is no data which has been published demonstrating that healthy people eating a well-balanced diet need any vitamin supplements." This opinion is shared by most physicians, not because of each physician's independent research of the data published on vitamins and minerals, but because of widespread physician ignorance in this area. For them, Dr. Herbert's blanket statement is the path of least resistance.

On the other hand there are claims that certain vitamins or minerals are all that are necessary to eliminate disease: Vitamin E prevents heart disease, they tell you. Selenium is for cancer, niacin for mental disorders. These proclamations are less respectable than the ordinary caution of the average family physician—but both represent medical error.

Dissension in medicine about supplements is real. It isn't a faked-up controversy such as the meat, egg, and dairy producers set up about the harm done by overeating fat, cholesterol, and protein. When I prescribe supplements I try to teach my patients how they work; I don't want them to wander out of the Institute and go on a supplements binge, believing supplements to be a wonderland of good health. I want them to use supplements intelligently and *not* just when they have become sick but in a way to promote health.

Let's look at how vitamins and minerals work in the body.

The Functions of Vitamins and Minerals

Genuine vitamins and minerals operate in the same way whether they are found in a leaf or in a bottle with the label of a reputable manufacturer on it. Here are the following ways they work:

**As co-enzymes.* I have mentioned enzymes before, especially those in the mouths of vegetable-eating animals that help to break down carbohydrates for use by the body. Enzymes do a number of jobs. They promote necessary reactions or changes in substances without being affected themselves. Instead of becoming part of a new substance to be absorbed, they affect the processing of food and are themselves eliminated. Therefore they have to be replaced or the next digestive job won't get done.

The body produces some complete enzymes. These do their work by themselves. Other body-produced substances are called apo-enzymes, and these become effectual only in the company of other substances that come into the body by mouth. Vitamins and minerals are needed to complete these enzymes, and when they work in this way we call them co-enzymes. Whether we obtain them from "natural" food or in tablet or capsule form, they work the same way. When they join an apo-enzyme the combination is ready to go to work, to effect a metabolic reaction.

**Independent affectors of metabolism.* Some vitamins and minerals work on their own to promote metabolic reactions without an apo-enzyme. For instance, vitamin D works like a hormone to regulate calcium metabolism.

Vitamin B_6 (Pyridoxine) sometimes acts as a co-enzyme and sometimes as an independent affector. A number of substances play dual or multiple roles in this way.

**Causes of deficiency.* A vitamin or mineral deficiency—lack of a needed substance demonstrated by marked symptoms of illness—is usually caused by an inadequacy of it in the person's food. The deficiency syndrome will take time to appear.

**A vitamin or mineral deficiency.* This lack of a needed substance is demonstrated by known symptoms of the illness and is usually caused by having too little of the substance in one's food. The deficiency syndrome will usually take some time to appear. A typical example: The symptoms of pellagra are the "three D's" of the ailment—dementia, dermatitis (skin eruption), and diarrhea.

**Hereditary defect.* Such a defect can prevent the body from producing a needed apo-enzyme. Then the normal intake of the potential co-enzyme will not be enough to benefit the system. A child born with inadequate production of the apo-enzyme methylmalonic isomerase, which normally binds to vitamin B_{12} to form a complete enzyme, will have severe mental retardation unless 1,000 mcg of B_{12} are ingested daily. But that dosage, which completely eliminates the problem, is 1,000 times the government's recommended daily allowance, or RDA. Which brings us to the trouble with the RDAs.

The Trouble with the RDAs

The Food and Nutrition Board of the National Academy of Sciences has issued guidelines about vitamin and mineral intake. In 1974 it stated that "the recommended dietary allowances are the levels of intake of essential nutrients considered, in the judgement of the Food and Nutrition Board, on the basis of available scientific knowledge, to be adequate to meet the known nutritional needs of practically all healthy persons."

Generally, studies on both human volunteers and animals are used to determine the RDAs. A clinical deficiency of a vitamin will be produced in a human volunteer or animal, and starting with very small doses of this vitamin, it is determined how much is needed to eliminate evidence of the deficiency. A modest increase is tacked onto this minimum amount for luck, and it becomes the standard RDA. There are three basic flaws in this method.

First, its aim is to eliminate a deficiency, and not to determine how much of a substance is needed to promote optimum health. A very small amount of a vitamin or mineral can eliminate evidence of gross deficiency. Larger amounts of these substances may stimulate production of much more of the enzyme in question, enough to improve the body's health from just off the danger list to excellent.

Riada Bayoumi and Sidney Rosalki, of St. Mary's Hospital in London, played some tricks on red blood cells taken from well-nourished individuals in whom no vitamin deficiency was suspected. To these red cells they added B_1, B_2, and B_6 vitamins, stimulating marked increases in enzyme production by the cells. If enzyme production by these cells had been at the maximum level, adding these vitamins would not have increased it. Did this indicate a mild if not a gross deficiency of the vitamins? Even if the blood donors did not seem ill-nourished?

The next step in this study was to supplement the diets of the subjects with B_1, B_2, and B_6 for seven days and then repeat the test with the addition of the vitamins to red cells in the lab. Much less enzyme was produced by the cells this time, indicating that the seven days of supplementation had saturated the enzyme system and brought it to a peak level.

These findings raise an obvious question. Is the best nutrition one stimulating top production of enzymes, or one that does no more than stimulate enough enzyme to eradicate symptoms of gross deficiency?

Another flaw in the way RDAs are established is that very arbitrary measurements are used. Only one effect of the vitamin is used to determine how much you should ingest. The test may have missed several other important effects of the vitamin on your health.

For instance, tiny amounts of vitamin C—5 to 10 mg daily—will eliminate signs of scurvy in guinea pigs. But 1,000 mg daily increases the mobility of white blood cells measurably, and increases production of interferon and of other immune globulins that are part of the body's defense against infection.

If we know that for a fact, how can we set the small amount of vitamin C needed to prevent scurvy as the recommended daily allowance, and warn people against taking more?

The way RDAs are established leaves out individual biological differences. What is enough for one person may be too little for the next. The differences between individual biological requirements are infinite. When one considers that vitamins are integrated into thousands of metabolic reactions, to assume that there are no inherent differences between individual needs defies reason.

Dr. Roger Williams, of the University of Texas and the Clayton Foundation, states that healthy people should use supplements as an "insurance formula" against possible deficiency. This does not mean that a deficiency will occur in the absence of the vitamin and mineral supplement, any more than not having fire insurance means that your house is going to burn down. But given the enormous potential for individual differences from person to person, and the varied mechanism of vitamin and mineral actions, supplementation seems to make sense.

Vitamin and Mineral Supplements in the Treatment of Disease

The prevailing concept of disease in medicine today is that individuals are normal until external vectors (germs, stress) cause disruption leading to disease. For instance, a virus infects normal cells, causing a cold. Until you had the cold you were clinically a well person. Everyone's constitution is supposedly strong, as strong as everyone else's, and those that break down do so because of external vectors.

Opposed to this is the concept of genetotrophic disease (*geneto* referring to genesis, *trophic* referring to feeding or nutrition). Dr. Roger Williams stated in 1950 that "partial genetic blocks lead to diminution but not complete failure of ability to carry out a specific enzymatic transformation, thereby increasing the need of the body for specific nutritional factor or factors." Simply stated, a genetotrophic disease develops in someone who is not getting enough of certain nutrients. The amount of these nutrients may be one hundred times the amount required by someone else, but without that much larger amount the individual is weakened and is more susceptible to disease: a cold, alcoholism, heart disease, cancer, etc.

The genetotrophic concept simply incorporates what we know to be obvious in biology, and what I have already mentioned, inherent differences between us as individuals. Just as no two oak leaves are identical, requirements for essential nutrients must be different among us as well. When the individual requirements are not met, disease occurs.

Finding a Genetotrophic Deficiency

Dr. D. Lonsdale and Dr. Raymond Shamberger, Department of Pediatrics, Cleveland Clinic, studied twenty patients, all of whom had various neurotic disorders which included depression, insomnia, irritability, chronic fatigue, nightmares, intermittent diarrhea and constipation, recurrent abdominal or chest pains. Elsewhere these patients would have received a battery of tests that turned up nothing, followed by psychotherapy and drugs to treat the symptoms.

These doctors went another way, looking for thiamin deficiency in the patients. They measured the transketolase activity in the red blood cells and found it to be low in twelve of the twenty patients. (Thiamin is the co-enzyme for producing the enzyme transketolase.) Diet histories showed that many of the patients were eating a lot of high-calorie foods such as carbonated sweet drinks and candy, in which the amount of vitamins and minerals per calorie is much lower than would be the case in unprocessed whole foods. Junk food calories have to be burned, and this calls for increased thiamin.

The twelve patients with low transketolase reactions were given a thiamin supplement ranging from 150 to 600 mg a day. These would be called megadoses, as the RDA for thiamin is only 1.2 mg for females and 1.6 mg for males. In all twelve patients the symptoms disappeared over a period of several weeks and the red blood cell transketolase reactions returned to normal.

You may ask, why not get those people off all the junk intake? That would probably have helped, but not with the discovery of the main thing that came out of the study. There was no measurable difference between the dietary patterns of the twelve patients with abnormal thiamin function and of the eight with normal thiamin function. Possibly the combination of the junk food with a larger genetic need for thiamin produced the deficiency that was reversed in the twelve.

Since the rest of the B complex vitamins, B_2, B_6, and pantothenic acid, also function as co-enzymes, it is possible that deficiencies of these could also produce the functional disturbances of insomnia, irritability, and a neurotic anxiety syndrome.

Mental Retardation: a Genetotrophic Disease?

Dr. Ruth H. Harrell, of Old Dominion University, Norfolk, Virginia, published in the *Proceedings of the National Academy of Science* in January, 1981, a study demonstrating that large doses of vitamins and minerals significantly increased the IQ in a group of mentally retarded children. She theorized that inadequate supplies of vitamins and minerals might have caused sluggish metabolism in the brains of the children. One group of children were given large doses of vitamin and mineral supplements and the other group got placebos. The children who got supplements showed a remarkable response. In four months they gained 9.6 in IQ, compared to a 1.1 gain for the control group. In the next four months the supplements-fed group gained another 6.2 points, making a total gain of 15.8 points in eight months. Meanwhile, the control group had been put on supplements at the end of the first four months, and at the end of the eight months they had gained 12.3 points. Several of the children were transferred to normal schools.

Besides the IQ increases there were improved growth rates. The children receiving the vitamins grew 2.13 centimeters in four months compared to .89 centimeters for the control group. All of these positive changes occurred without a single negative side effect.

A Word of Warning

I am about to go into some of the benefits of individual supplements, and I always feel uncomfortable about doing this because I *don't* want to make any supplement seem to be a magic cure by itself. No vitamin or mineral is The Answer. One reason I want to have a patient at the Institute for twelve days is to inculcate in him or her that a total program—diet, exercise, supplements, oxygen—is needed to reverse heart disease. As helpful as supplements are, they may be wasted if not integrated into a complete program. But, since I have questioned the RDAs as guidelines, I think I must show the effects of vitamins and minerals in doses exceeding the RDAs.

Vitamins E and C and Selenium as Antioxidants

The cells need oxygen, but oxidation of cell constituents is harmful and comes of contact, not with oxygen, but with certain substances called free radicals. Exposure to free radicals is unavoidable, but the body has mechanisms to control oxidation and these can be aided by taking the antioxidant vitamins E and C, and the mineral selenium.

Free radicals are highly reactive substances that oxidize cell constituents, particularly unsaturated fat molecules. Once oxidized, these fat molecules become free radicals themselves, so that the oxidation process becomes a chain reaction.

Some common free radicals are atmospheric pollutants like ozone, drugs like carbon tetrachloride, paraquat, and adriamycin. Many commonly eaten foods contain free radicals. Cholesterol exposed to heat and oxygen together, as in the frying pan, can oxidize and become a free radical.

Vitamins E and C are antioxidants in themselves, and selenium fights oxidation as part of a selenium-dependent enzyme, glutathione peroxidase.

There are three ways by which cells are protected from the oxidizing free radicals.

*Antioxidants and antioxidant enzyme systems preferentially soak up free radicals and neutralize them before they damage normal cells. Vitamins E and C have this function.

*Certain antioxidants, including vitamins E and C, prevent free radicals from forming. This is why vitamin C is often added to foodstuffs to prolong shelf life. Spoilage is generally the production of free radicals by oxidation. Two other commonly used food additives, BHT and BHA, are also antioxidants.

*The membrane of cells can be strengthened against attack by free radicals. Several nutrients strengthen the membranes but vitamins E and C and selenium are particularly needed.

Dr. Daniel Menzen, of the University of California at Davis, kept rats in a high-ozone atmosphere; some of them were fed vitamin E and others denied it. The deprived rats lived eight days. Those on vitamin E lived ten days longer. The dosage of vitamin E needed to protect the lungs against ozone is much higher than what is generally considered adequate.

Additional Benefits of Vitamins C and E

**Effects on blood cholesterol.* Some studies show definite changes in blood cholesterol after taking vitamin C, but there is conflicting evidence. Dr. Ginter, Institute of Human Nutrition Research, Czechoslovakia, gave eighty-two men one gram of vitamin C daily. He noted significant blood cholesterol drops, especially in those with levels above 230. In nineteen subjects whose average cholesterol level was 260, the average level fell to 220. This effect may be due to vitamin C's influence on the transformation of cholesterol in the liver into bile acid, which is then excreted through the intestinal tract.

Dr. L.K. Kothari, of Medical College of Udaipur, India, found that one gram of vitamin C taken daily for one month lowered the cholesterol level in ten young men from 204 to 177 and in ten middle-aged men from 256 to 225. Other studies, however, have not confirmed a significant or predictable lowering of the blood cholesterol level with vitamin C.

**Vitamin C thins the blood.* As blood rushes through arteries roughened by cholesterol plaque, a clot can form plugging the artery and causing a heart attack. Dr. Constance Leslie found that one gram of vitamin C reduced the chances of an abnormal clot by 50 percent. Dr. K.E. Sarji, Veteran's Hospital of South Carolina Medical Center, found that four grams of vitamin C daily significantly decreased the aggregation or stickiness of platelets in diabetic patients, and two grams decreased the aggregation of platelets in normal men.

**Vitamin C protects artery linings.* Perhaps the most important benefit is the protective effect of vitamin C on the lining of the artery.

Dr. G.C. Willis, a Canadian, demonstrated this with a group of guinea pigs. Deprived of vitamin C, they developed scurvy and atherosclerosis. When vitamin C was added to their diet the atherosclerosis was reversed.

Dr. F.J. Finamore, of the Biology Division of Oakridge National Laboratory, studied rabbits on a high-fat, high-cholesterol diet. The rabbits who did not receive vitamin C developed 250 percent more cholesterol deposits in the arteries than those who got the vitamin C. Vitamin C apparently makes the lining more resistant to the kind of injury that permits plaque formation.

**Vitamin E thins the blood.* Perhaps even more than vitamin C, vitamin E tends to prevent abnormal blood clotting. In one study of ten diabetic patients, vitamin E reduced the clumping of platelets. Several physicians have reported using this vitamin to prevent pulmonary embolus (a clot that travels to the lung) after surgery.

**Vitamin E increases HDL cholesterol.* Several reports have shown that vitamin E increases the beneficial HDL fraction of cholesterol in patients who have low HDL levels. Dr. William J. Hermann at Morrow City General Hospital, Houston, reported an increase in HDL and a reduction in the low-density cholesterol and triglycerides. Dr. Joseph J. Baborikrik, of the Wisconsin Veterans Administration Medical Center in Milwaukee, reported increased HDL cholesterol in forty-three subjects who had had low levels after only four weeks of taking vitamin E.

**Vitamin E helps angina.* Although many studies have not demonstrated that vitamin E is significant in the treatment of angina, in one study reported by Dr. D.V. Frost and Dr. P.M. Lish, one milligram of selenium plus 200 units of vitamin E were shown to offer significant clinical benefit in angina. Twenty-two out of twenty-four patients were judged to have benefited during the treatment period, while only five out of twenty-four who received placebo showed any benefit.

**Vitamin E improves intermittent claudication.* Pain in the legs with walking, called intermittent claudication, is similar to angina or heart pain. It is brought on by exercise. When one walks, the muscles of the legs require more oxygen than they can get when the arteries are clogged; this increased oxygen can't be delivered and the muscles begin to ache. Vitamin E has been shown to reduce leg pain and increase exercise tolerance. Dr. Knut Haeger, Slotts-

Staden Clinic, Sweden, in a sixteen-year study, reported beneficial results using vitamin E. Improvement was slow; it took eighteen months before a difference could be shown between recipients and a control group. Other studies bear out this finding. Most researchers agree that it takes three months or more on vitamin E before improvement can be noted.

Chromium

As early as 1854 it was reported that brewer's yeast improved the diabetic condition. The active ingredient found in brewer's yeast was a complex of chromium and several amino acids called glucose tolerance factor. Dr. Walter Mertz, at the Walter Reed Army Institute of Research, found that a chromium supplement improved diabetic control in three out of six diabetics. The glucose tolerance factor does not act like insulin; it seems to potentiate the function of insulin, allowing for more efficient blood sugar control. The concentration of chromium in the tissues of Americans declines with age, and Dr. Mertz speculates that this chromium deficiency plays a role in the onset of diabetes later in life. He also noted that the positive response to chromium supplementation may take as long as three months.

Chromium deficiency is also related to atherosclerosis. Dr. Henry Schroeder, of Dartmouth Medical School, found that chromium deficiency in rats would cause diabetes, high blood cholesterol, and accelerated atherosclerosis, while chromium supplementation would prevent these conditions. He also reported that chromium concentration was deficient in the aortas of patients dying from atherosclerotic heart disease, whereas this concentration was normal in patients without severe atherosclerosis.

Dr. Howard A. Newman, Ohio State University, found that patients with positive angiograms for coronary artery disease had "... significantly lower serum chromium concentration than did the group with normally patent [open] arteries."

In a recent study by Dr. S.A. Abraham, of Hebrew University Medical School, Israel, supplemental chromium was found to accelerate the reversal of atherosclerosis in rabbits. Twenty-three rabbits were established in reversal of atherosclerosis by going on a low-fat diet; of these, twelve were also given daily chromium in small doses. The chromium-fed rabbits showed much greater reversal than the control group.

Dr. J.C. Elwood tested effects of chromium-rich yeast products on eleven volunteers with normal blood lipids and sixteen with elevated blood lipids. For eight weeks both groups got twenty grams daily of brewer's yeast containing forty-eight micrograms of chromium. Cholesterol levels dropped and HDL went up significantly in both groups.

At the Institute we use a yeast grown on a chromium-rich medium that increases the trivalent chromium content to one hundred times that present in brewer's yeast. One level teaspoon contains about 200 mcg of chromium. Patients take one teaspoon daily.

Betty K. is a good example of how this form of chromium can produce results. She came to us with diabetes, high blood pressure, and mild heart disease. At the time she entered we were not using the high-chromium yeast, and her results, though improved, were not satisfactory to either of us. In two weeks her cholesterol dropped from 241 to 215, her blood sugar from 211 to 188, and triglycerides went up from 262 to 278. She continued the diet at home for a month but a follow-up test showed cholesterol 247, sugar 195, and triglycerides 508. A daily dose of 600 mcg of the high-chromium yeast was added to her diet. In three weeks her cholesterol was 168, sugar 86, and triglycerides 116.

Gamma Linolenic Acid

Lowering fat intake is of paramount importance, but some fats are essential, and this is one of the most valuable supplements. Linoleic acid, an unsaturated fat, is essential to health; it should make up at least 1 percent of caloric intake.

Linoleic acid does little by itself until it is converted by the body into gamma linolenic acid and then into a group of hormones called the prostaglandins, which have beneficial effect on the blood cholesterol activity of insulin, blood pressure, stickiness of the blood, arthritis, and even the patient's mood. The prostaglandins have been the subject of intense medical study over the last ten years.

Low activity or absence of an enzyme, Delta-6 desaturase, reduces the conversion of linoleic acid to gamma linolenic acid, thus reducing the amount of the beneficial circulating prostaglandins. Taking vegetable oils rich in linoleic acid in the absence of the Delta-6 desaturase has limited effect. If we could take the gamma linolenic acid by mouth we could bystep the rate-limiting Delta-6—but there are only two food sources of this acid.

One is mother's milk. For most of us this is an impractical source. Another is the oil of the evening primrose, which is about 9 percent gamma linolenic acid. Dr. David Horrobin found that small amounts of this supplement caused marked drops in blood cholesterol, especially in people with high cholesterol levels. He has done controlled studies on over 2,000 patients, and these show that the supplement may play a role in lowering blood pressure, lowering and reducing insulin requirements, and depression. More studies are needed to define exactly how this unique vegetable oil works in our body.

Eicosapentaenoic Acid

This is the component of marine mammal fat and fish oil that is so helpful in the Eskimo diet. Like gamma linolenic acid, it lowers the cholesterol level. Dr. Scott Goodnight and Dr. W.E. Connor, at the University of Oregon, fed ten volunteers a diet of mostly salmon fillets for four weeks. He noted a 17 percent drop in cholesterol and a 40 percent drop in triglycerides. He also measured the effect of the salmon oil on platelet function. Platelets are small, sand-like particles, flowing in the blood, that function as clotting agents. When a vessel is damaged (as in a small cut), platelets adhere to the injury and initiate clot formation.

Platelets can also initiate and accelerate atherosclerosis. When they adhere abnormally to artery walls they release a growth factor that stimulates cell division in the smooth muscle cells of the artery wall, and this initiates atherosclerosis. Also, if they adhere to a plaque, they can form an abnormal clot which can block off a vessel and cause a heart attack or a stroke.

In those volunteers eating the salmon fillets, the platelet count was reduced 40 percent and the platelets were less sticky (and therefore less prone to adhere to the wall of an artery). So it seems that a diet rich in marine oils would have a two-fold protective effect. It would lower the blood fats—triglycerides even more than cholesterol—and it would have an antithrombotic action on platelets.

Most Americans refuse a daily diet of fish. Those volunteers got sick of salmon fillets—they sound mouth-watering until you've eaten them for a solid week. And, of course, there is the high cost of seafood now. But fish oil, rich in eicosapentaenoic acid, is available in one-gram capsules, and we routinely give them to patients at the Institute.

Questions Patients Ask Me

I have patients who have long been dosing themselves with supplements, and reading popular tracts on the subject. They come to me loaded with strong opinions on the subject. And I have others who have a strong prejudice against any nutrients that come from a drugstore. Both sorts ask questions, and certain questions come up again and again. I would like to answer a number of these here.

**Are natural vitamins better than synthetic?*

I'm afraid not. The genuine vitamin, whether found in a vegetable food or synthesized in a lab, is always the same substance. You can bet that any tablet with a significant amount of any vitamin is largely synthetic. There is deception in a great deal of vitamin labeling. In a bottle of vitamin C labeled "With Rose Hips," most of the vitamin is of synthetic origin. This is legal, since the maker says "with" and not "all." And he can add "All Natural" to his label, because any substance normally occurring in the body, whether of plant, animal, or synthetic origin, is considered to be natural. If a manufacturer adds some rose hip or acerola powder to his vitamin C, he is not required to say how much, because chemically this is immaterial.

Rose hip powder contains vitamin C, but not much. In one analysis it was found to have 25 mg of ascorbic acid in 100,000 mg of rose hip powder. A tablet containing 250 mg of vitamin C derived solely from rose hip powder would be the size of a basketball.

One gram of dried whole liver contains .05 mg of B_{12}, .25 mg of niacin, and smaller amounts of other B complex factors. Tablets of this "natural" substance have to contain synthetically derived preparations of the vitamin.

If you pay extra for "natural" supplements you are paying for the label.

**Don't "natural" vitamin preparations contain substances, other than the vitamin, that are of value, that help the vitamin to do its work?*

No. Any other substance of value should be obtained in whole natural foods.

**Can vitamins and minerals be toxic in large doses?*

The vitamins most likely to be toxic are the fat-soluble ones. A and D carry the most risk. Vitamin E in excessive doses may be toxic. These fat-soluble vitamins are stored in the fat tissues of the body, and an excess can't be eliminated. For this reason we never prescribe more of these than is present in our supplement formula.

Trace minerals are potentially toxic, too. They may upset the balance of mineral metabolism as well as having specific toxicity. Therefore, we keep our trace mineral supplement program within general prescribed levels of these minerals and give them in a balanced formula. Again, we are trying to de-emphasize the concept of taking a specific mineral, or vitamin for that matter, for a specific problem.

The water-soluble B complex and vitamin C are non-toxic. After saturating the system, the excess amounts of these substances are generally eliminated from the body in the urine. There was a report just recently of five women who took very large doses of B_6 by itself, ranging between 2,000 and 5,000 mg a day. This was done on the inaccurate assumption that the B_6 would serve as a diuretic. These individuals experienced weakness and loss of sensation as a result of damage to the peripheral nerves primarily in the lower extremity. These symptoms abated with cessation of the high B_6 intake. It is interesting that this report received wide publicity on the toxicity of vitamin B_6 but little mention was made of the very high and excessive doses of B_6 being used by these individuals. For instance, our recommendation of B_6 is only 1/20 of the amount that brings on the symptoms and no toxicity to my knowledge has been recorded with a B_6 intake in the range of 50–200 mg per day. To illustrate the very significant safety record of the water-soluble vitamins, consider what would happen to you if you took twenty times the average dose of aspirin, going from two tablets every four hours to forty tablets every four hours. Or, for that matter, consider what would happen should you take twenty times the therapeutic dose of any prescription drug, on a regular basis.

In some cases inaccurate information has been disseminated about the toxicity of certain vitamins. A prime example is the rather widespread belief that large amounts of vitamin C inactivate B_{12} and would perhaps cause a B_{12} deficiency. In 1974 Dr. Victor Herbert published a study in which he took 500 mg of vitamin C and incubated this with a standard meal of known B_{12} concentration. When he measured the B_{12} concentration before and after the incubation he apparently found that some of the B_{12} had been inactivated. He concluded his study with the statement, "high doses of vitamin C, popularly used as a home remedy against the common cold, destroy substantial amounts of B_{12} when ingested with food. . . . Daily ingestion of 500 mgs. or more of ascorbic acid without regular evaluation of B_{12} status is probably unwise." Since publication of this article his closing statement has been repeated in many nutrition-related articles.

Unfortunately, the methods used by Dr. Herbert to measure B_{12} in the meal both before and after vitamin C were grossly inaccurate. In fact, his method of measurement accounted only for a fraction of the vitamin B_{12} that was actually present. His study was repeated by Dr. H.L. Newmark, this time using accurate measurements of vitamin B_{12}. Dr. Newmark found that the actual amount of B_{12} present in the test meals was six to eight times that reported by Dr. Herbert and that the addition of 100 mg, 250 mg, or 500 mg of ascorbic acid led to no change in the amount of B_{12} in the meal. We can therefore conclude that the hazard ascribed to the intake with meals of moderately large amounts of vitamin C, 500 mg or more, does not exist.

Another erroneous belief goes back to a Food and Drug Administration warning that vitamin C might cause kidney stones. The FDA had no evidence to back this up—only an indication that vitamin C could possibly elevate oxalic acid in the blood and urine. When Linus Pauling asked the FDA to defend its stand it could not.

Neither the B_{12} deficiency nor the kidney-stone theory is borne out by any incident in a population in which millions of people take vitamin C supplements. Nobody has been reported as having developed a B_{12} deficiency that way. No definite connection between vitamin C and kidney stones has been made to my knowledge.

I would never say that there is no danger of toxicity in vitamin and mineral supplements. But at this writing, taken in the doses that are recommended, I am not aware of any significant danger or side effect having been reported.

The Rationale for the Supplement Program

Dosages of supplements at the Institute are somewhat arbitrary. There is no technology for assessing the optimum level of each nutrient for each patient. What we do is supply substantial amounts of all the water-soluble nutrients, since these have little or no toxicity, any excess being freely eliminated by the body. We use smaller doses of the fat-soluble vitamins E, A, and D, since these are stored in the body fat and have a higher potential for toxicity.

The aim of our nutrient supplement program is to saturate the enzyme systems with the hope of eliminating genetotropic dysfunction, the inborn inability to utilize food to the body's best advantage.

Certain supplements are increased to achieve a specific purpose. This is done on an individual basis, and with close monitoring. The formula for our general vitamin and mineral program is below. This program is provided to the patients at the Institute and when they leave they receive a multiple preparation that complies with formulation. In addition we have our patients taking on the average one gram of evening primrose oil per meal and two to three grams of Max EPA fish oil per meal.

For more information about availability of this formulation of vitamins and minerals please contact the Institute.

	Amount	%USRDA
Vitamin A (beta carotene)	20,000 IU	400
Vitamin B_1 (thiamin-HCL)	10 mg	667
Vitamin B_2 (riboflavin)	10 mg	588
Niacinamide	100 mg	500
Pantothenic Acid (Ca pantothenate)	50 mg	500
Vitamin B_6 (pyridoxine-HCL)	50 mg	2,500
Vitamin B_{12} (cyanocobalamin)	30 mcg	500
Folic Acid	400 mcg	100
Biotin	100 mcg	*
Vitamin C (ascorbic acid)	1,000 mg	1,667

	Amount	%USRDA
Vitamin D (ergocalciferol)	400 IU	100
Vitamin E (d-alpha-tocopheryl acetate)	400 IU	1,333
Choline (bitartrate)	1,000 mg	*
Calcium (carbonate)	1,000 mg	100
Magnesium (oxide)	400 mg	100
Zinc (gluconate)	30 mg	200
Iron (ferrous fumarate)	18 mg	100
Manganese (gluconate)	10 mg	*
Copper (gluconate)	2 mg	100
Selenium (Nutrition 21 yeast)	200 mcg	*
Chromium (Chromax-GTF)	100 mcg	*
Iodine (KI)	150 mcg	100
Molybdenum (sodium molybdate)	50 mg	*
Silicon (magnesium trisilicate)	20 mg	*
Potassium (chloride)	860 mg	*

*No USRDA established.

14

Exercise for a Healthy Heart

Imagine sitting in your doctor's office. He hesitates, then says, "My friend, I'm going to write you a prescription that will make you feel better, help you to lose weight, eliminate insomnia, reduce stress and anxiety, curb your appetite, improve your creativity, tone your muscles, improve your self-image, increase your confidence, protect you from a heart attack and diabetes, slow down about every 'measurement of the aging process,' and regardless of how you feel now, will make you feel better."

"Wonderful," you say, "but that must cost a lot."

"No, it's free except for about thirty to forty-five minutes of your time four times a week. It's exercise."

The exercise boom is on. Check out the parks, the high school track, the racquetball courts, the bike paths: literally millions of people have discovered what exercise can do, and are busy reaping the benefits. The only negative comments about exercise seem to come from those who don't.

The rebirth of exercise is truly remarkable and comes just in time. The comforts of technology were close to eliminating our need for any movement at all. With the advent of technology evolved a culture of "brains," with no need for using muscle or bones. Then it happened, people began running around again—just for the fun of it. Just fifteen years ago, only a few hundred "weirdos" lined up to run the Boston marathon of twenty-six continuous miles. That event now attracts about 5,000 who must meet exceedingly difficult standards to qualify. The New York Marathon is fifteen years old, yet attracts 17,000 runners. The Bay to the Breakers race through the streets of San Francisco attracted about a thousand entrants in the midsixties. Today, over 60,000 cover the seven and a half–mile course and it's a West Coast happening.

This physical fitness fervor is perhaps a major reason that death from heart disease has declined over the last fifteen years. While exercise is not "the answer," it surely seems to prevent heart disease.

What Type of Exercise?

The only type of exercise that builds the kind of health we're talking about is aerobic or isotonic exercise. This includes such activities as walking, jogging, racquetball, bicycling, and swimming, all which cause the heart to beat faster, the lungs to bring in more air, and an increase of oxygen to muscles and the heart. Generally the best indicator of the degree of exercise is the heart rate, which goes up with aerobic exercise.

Another form of exercise is anaerobic, or isometric, which includes weight lifting, many of the popular Nautilus exercise routines, and true isometric tension maneuvers against an immovable bar. These exercises increase tone and bulk of muscle, but do not condition the heart. In fact, lifting heavy weights or true isometric exercise causes an increase in blood pressure which can be dangerous.

A third form of exercise practiced by many is the stretching done in yoga along with deep breathing maneuvers. While these activities can be very pleasant and imbue a sense of tranquility and calm, they do not strengthen the heart or improve its function. Therefore, the only form of exercise to be discussed here is the aerobic, for it is this type that is essential in treating and preventing heart disease. Yet it does so much more that we should exercise regularly even if heart disease were not evident.

A Mood Elevator

As a group, you may find runners to be arrogant, humble, opinionated, flexible, pushy, courteous, loud, or soft-spoken. But you don't find them to be depressed. In fact, regular physical exercise and depression are virtually incompatible, so much so that several psychiatrists and psychologists now prescribe running for emotional disturbances. Dr. Thadius Costrabala, a psychiatrist in the San Diego area, conducts group and individual therapy sessions while jogging along the beach.

Dr. John H. Greist, Professor of Psychiatry at the University of Wisconsin, studied a group of depressed patients, as determined by the SCL-90 depression test, and divided them into three different groups. Eight patients received no therapy, but were enrolled in a jogging program. Seven patients received a time-structured (fifty minutes) behavior modification therapy, and nine patients received insight-oriented therapy with no time restrictions.

The test ran for twelve weeks. The results: The runners fared the best. Six out of eight lost their depression completely and the average scores of the group at the end demonstrated almost no depression. The time-structured group with the behavior modification approach were next, but their scores started to deteriorate during the last weeks of the study, possibly as they contemplated having to live without the therapy. Those with unlimited therapy sessions had the worst results being more depressed at the end of the twelve weeks than before they started.

How could jogging succeed where therapy failed? Mood is structured by a complex hormone balance in the brain; one is noradrenaline, also called norepinephrine. Many of the anti-depressant drugs elevate mood by increasing the amount of this hormone in the brain. Exercise literally floods the entire body with noradrenaline, consequently lifting depression.

Depression is a serious problem, affecting at least 10 percent of the population chronically. Of course we all have depression to some degree, at some time. In fact, many people are mildly depressed all the time yet function adequately. These people simply don't experience life as "fun" or "exciting." But exercise can change that. In one study of sixty-seven "normal" college professors, eleven (16 percent) measured in the depressed range when given a standardized test. All participated in a six-week program of aerobic exercise three times a week. Afterward the eleven "depressed" professors were no longer depressed, nor were any of the other participants. Only aerobic exercise confers this elevated mood. In another study, 167 college students signed up for various physical activities which included softball, wrestling, tennis, or jogging. They also took before and after standardized depression scores. The joggers showed the greatest improvement in depression, the softball players and six students who didn't exercise showed the least. It is the aerobic exercise which increases the heart rate that does the trick.

Even more exciting than noradrenaline is a newly discovered hormone called beta endorphine. This is produced by the brain and has a marked effect on mood, sense of well-being, and pain. In fact, the powerful painkillers like morphine and Demerol work by enhancing the endorphine system to relieve pain and produce a sense of well-being. Beta endorphine activates the pleasure centers in the brain, and in a real sense is a chemical explanation of optimism, positive self-image, and that elusive "sense of well-being."

Walter M. Bortz, II, M.D., from Stanford University School of Medicine, measured norepinephrine and B-endorphine levels in several well-trained athletes before, during, and after a particularly grueling race of, would you believe, one hundred miles; the winner finished in eighteen hours and thirty-five minutes! To qualify for entry, each participant had to have completed a fifty-mile race. The norepinephrine and B-endorphine levels before the race were higher than the laboratory's normal values and went up markedly during and after the race. They were, in fact, the highest levels ever recorded by that laboratory.

No doubt about it; exercise stirs up the hormones and increases the sum total of everything good—happiness—and you don't need to run one hundred miles. Other studies have shown that brisk walking, or bike riding, for fifteen to twenty-five minutes will make the difference.

Just how "happy" are you, anyway? Would you describe yourself as (1) very happy, (2) pretty happy, or (3) not too happy? Dr. Richard Carter, a psychiatrist resident at the University of Washington, asked 216 adults the same questions and correlated their responses to their exercise habits. He found a direct association between happiness and physical fitness. For instance, of those who responded "very happy" 72.1 percent got enough exercise to be classed as physically fit, while only 37.7 percent of the "pretty happy" group and 35.3 percent of the "not so happy" group were physically fit.

Exercise makes you feel good, enlivening your experience of life, which is why so many people do it! Those people running around in the park, and on the bike paths, are not trying to prevent a heart attack (even though it does). They do it because they feel better, and modern science, with its sophisticated hormone measurements, confirms what they already knew: Life is vibrant if lived actively, and dull if lived inactively.

"But doctor," you might say, "I always feel good—and I never exercise!"

To that I reply, "Do you know what you're missing?" I remember a case of a young eighteen-year-old girl who for most of her life had a severe case of undiagnosed anemia (low blood level). When it was discovered, the doctors kept asking her if she had been feeling tired and she said no. Not until her severe anemia had been corrected did she understand what the doctors meant; she had been chronically fatigued for so long that to her it was "natural."

It is safe to say that exercise will make you feel better; if you feel bad, you'll feel good, if you feel good, you'll feel better. That is reason enough for you to start, but now let's see what exercise does for healthy and unhealthy hearts.

Exercise and Heart Failure

It all started in 1953. Professor Jeremy Morris, of the British Medical Research Council, published a study of death rates among the bus drivers and bus conductors of the London Transport Department. The paper, entitled "Coronary Heart Disease and Physical Activity at Work," reported that conductors of the buses had one-third less heart disease than the drivers, and only one-half the number of fatal and non-fatal heart attacks. The reason? Exercise!

As you probably know, most buses in London are double-decker, and the conductors' job was fare collection from each passenger. While the driver was sitting, the conductor was constantly active going up and down the stairs and down the aisles twenty-four times an hour. This is equivalent to climbing up and down the stairs of an average two-story home a hundred times a day!

Dr. Morris pointed out that the reduced death rate of the conductors could be due to other causes, but his observations opened everyone's eyes to the potential value of exercise and further studies quickly followed. One such study revealed that among postal workers, those who delivered the mail on foot had only one-half the heart problems as those who sorted the mail. Another study showed that active railroad switchmen had only one-third the heart problems as sedentary ticket clerks. In every large study of workers, those whose jobs were active had only one-third to one-half the heart problems compared to those whose jobs were sedentary.

Dr. Daniel Bruner from Israel had a unique opportunity to study people living in the Israeli kibbutz, where the environment and diet were uniform. When settling in Israel, many Jewish immigrants chose to live "in community" where all the facilities were shared by everyone, and there were no discrepancies in the standard of living regardless of occupation. For instance, all the meals for the community were prepared by those whose task was food service, while others either worked in the fields, did the carpentry and building, took care of the children, did the clerical work, etc. Dr. Bruner found that heart disease was 2.5 to 4.0 times greater in the sedentary workers than in the active workers.

"But doctor," you may lament, "I'm not a postman, or a bus conductor. My job requires that I sit at a desk for eight hours a day!"

We do live in an advanced society in which almost all physical effort has been removed from work. This is great. Unlike many who write about exercise and wish for a return to the days of hard physical labor, I relish the modern conveniences and comforts brought on by technology. The work-saving advances of modern life have liberated all of us to create, express, and live like no other culture in human history. In fact, when we consider the comforts and conveniences that we take for granted even the poor among us live like kings of years gone by. We have hot and cold running water (no more need to lug water from the well), instant communication with telephones (no more jogging into town to see so-and-so), instant entertainment from television (we are now spectators, seldom participants), stoves that provide heat by simply turning a switch (when was the last time you chopped, stacked, and hauled wood?), and automobiles or buses for transportation (how many pairs of walking shoes do you wear out each year?).

Are these advances bad? Not necessarily, for they have also given us free time, and *active* free time confers the same protection against heart disease as does active work. In 1973, twenty years after his landmark study of the bus conductors, Dr. Morris published a study of the leisure time activities of 17,000 British civil servants. He found that those whose non-work activities were vigorous, such as brisk walking, swimming, bicycling, or soccer for thirty minutes a day had only one-third the heart problems of those whose leisure activities were sedentary. He also found that the more vigorous the exercise, the lower were the instances of heart problems. He concluded that "...habitual vigorous exercise during leisure time reduces the instances of coronary heart disease...." and that "...training of the heart and cardiovascular system is one of the mechanisms of protection...." Dr. Ralph S. Paffenbarger, Jr., Professor of Epidemiology at Stanford University School of Medicine, was able to quantify various activities in terms of calories of energy expenditure. For instance, climbing one flight of stairs once a day per week expends 28 calories, while one city block of walking per day expends 56 calories in a week. Light sports burn 5 calories per minute, and strenuous sports burn 10 calories per minute. He surveyed 17,000 Harvard graduates, and with a questionnaire was able to quantify the degree of activity each expended during a regular week. He then divided men into three groups based upon the amount of calories expended in activity and found that the sedentary group who expended fewer than 500 calories a week had a heart attack rate of 70.7 per 10,000 man years of observation. The middle group expended between 500 and 1,999 calories a week in exercise and had a heart attack rate of 53.3, while the active group who expended more than 2,000 calories a week had a heart attack rate of only 35.3. The difference between the active and sedentary groups was over 50 percent. Taken as a whole, the studies unequivocally show that regular exercise will reduce the risk of heart disease from 30 to 60 percent. Dr. Paffenbarger, a strong believer in his own study, ran seventy-nine miles in one week before the 50th Annual Scientific Session of the American Heart Association. While you need not run nearly eighty miles in one week, you can spend more than 2,000 calories a week in exercise by averaging only thirty minutes a day in brisk walking, swimming, bicycling, or slow jogging. How does exercise work?

1. Exercise Conditions the Heart

Regular exercise causes a sustained measurable increase in the function of the heart. It (a) increases the efficiency of oxygen utilization by the heart, as well as other muscles. This means that a conditioned heart can extract more oxygen from a given amount of blood than an unconditioned heart and (b) as we begin to age, our capacity to utilize large amounts of oxygen goes down. However, regular physical exercise can give a person sixty years old the same maximum oxygen utilization as someone forty years old.

Like any muscle, the heart becomes stronger with regular use.

The conditioned heart is able to pump more blood with each beat than the unconditioned heart. This reduces the workload of the heart and the resting heart rate drops. One of the earliest measurable changes to occur with exercise is a slower pulse rate at rest. For instance, the average pulse rate of an unconditioned heart at rest would be about 75 to 85 beats per minute. After several weeks of exercise, the heart rate indicates the more efficient extraction of oxygen as well as the increased strength of the heart muscle. In short, the heart is working less and working more efficiently. Since the unconditioned heart is beating an average of 20 beats more per minute, these extra beats quickly add up. That's 12,000 additional beats per hour, 288,000 additional beats per day, and 9,137,600 additional beats per year.

The slower the heartbeat the greater the blood flow in the heart arteries. The heart receives blood only between beats, because the valves that allow blood to flow to the heart muscle are closed when the heart contracts to pump blood. But, they open again when the heart is relaxed in the resting phase of its cycle. Since the conditioned heart has a much longer rest period, more blood is able to flow to the heart muscle.

2. Exercise Improves the Blood Lipids and Thins the Blood

Exercise does not significantly lower the blood cholesterol level—only diet can do that—but it does alter the low-density and high-density cholesterol fractions. As we discussed earlier, cholesterol that is carried in a complex with protein, called high-density cholesterol, is protective while cholesterol that is carried in a fat complex, called low-density cholesterol, rips into the arteries and causes plaques. Numerous studies have shown that habitual aerobic exercise elevates the HDL cholesterol and lowers the LDL cholesterol. In addition, exercise lowers the triglyceride or circulating fat as well.

Often heart attacks occur when blood flowing over roughened and diseased arteries forms a clot which totally blocks the blood flow into the artery. Blood normally clots when you injure yourself, whether it be a cut on your finger or a sprained ankle. Obviously this clotting mechanism is a wonderful protective phenomenon, for we are well aware of the problems that beset a "bleeder" who has an abnormal clotting mechanism. However, when clots form inside the arteries, this can be disastrous. The body has its own protective mechanism for avoiding this abnormal clot formation, which is called fibrinolysis. Basically, it is a system of rapidly acting enzymes that immediately dissolve small abnormal clots before they are able to block the arteries. Numerous studies have shown that regular exercise activates this system and protects the heart and other organs from abnormal clot formation.

3. Exercise Enlarges Heart Arteries

When Clarence DeMar, a famous long-distance runner, died of cancer at the age of seventy-two, an autopsy revealed that his heart arteries were much larger than normal. This was surely a direct result of his many years of vigorous exercise. A study in the December 1981 issue of the *New England Journal of Medicine* by Dieter M. Kramsch showed that monkeys who were given a high-fat, high-cholesterol diet, yet exercised on a treadmill for one hour, three times a week, showed marked reduction in the degree of atherosclerosis in the arteries, enlargement of the arteries to the heart, and a compensatory enlargement of the heart itself which is also seen in healthy athletes. He succinctly concluded that "... the benefits derived from such moderate exercise for one hour, three times per week in the presence of hypercholesterolemia (high blood cholesterol as a result of the diet), were less atherosclerosis in wider coronary arteries supplying a larger heart that functioned at a slower rate."

4. Exercise Increases Collateral Arteries

When the arteries to the heart or any other organ begin to close down, the body starts to build new arteries that travel around the blockage. This natural bypass is called "collateral circulation" and has been life-saving in millions of men and women. Often angiograms, which are special x-rays of the heart arteries, demonstrate that a major heart artery has closed completely, but the person was spared a heart attack by collaterals which sprung up in other sections of the heart to protect that section in jeopardy. In a sense there is a race between the closing of the artery and the development of collateral arteries: if closure wins, you could die; if the collateralization wins, you may be spared. Numerous studies on dogs, monkeys, and other animals have shown that exercise accelerates the development of collaterals when the major arteries are closing. In fact, exercise is the only variable that will accelerate collateral development.

But, in this race between closure and collateral development, the stakes are too high for you to lose, because you could lose everything. The purpose of this book is to inform you about a dietary program which can stop and reverse the atherosclerosis, while you utilize exercise to protect and condition the heart, as well as build collaterals.

When Jim Fixx, the author of *The Complete Book of Running,* died while jogging, again the safety of jogging was discussed in the front pages of our nation's newspapers. Those in favor of exercise were not budging from their position that exercise on the whole was safe and beneficial, while those that had criticized the exercise boom increased their attacks on the proponents' claims. What interested me about this dialogue was the almost complete absence of any discussion of diet or, even more specifically, the blood cholesterol level of Jim Fixx. Only one newspaper article carried the account that Mr. Fixx rarely saw a physician and that his last blood cholesterol level was 254, which, in my opinion, is way too high and consistent with untimely death from cardiovascular disease. Also, Mr. Fixx's father died at a very early age from heart disease—forty-four—which indicates an inherited tendency toward elevated cholesterol. The fact that Jim Fixx lived to his midfifties could be viewed as a positive result of vigorous exercise.

Be that as it may, I would like to state clearly my personal view of the role of exercise in the prevention of heart disease.

1. Our high-fat, high-cholesterol diet—not lack of exercise—is the major culprit when it comes to producing heart disease and causing untimely death. Untimely death will occur even in the well-conditioned if the blood cholesterol level remains high.
2. Exercise does condition the heart and does confer protection from heart disease, but it in no way guarantees immunity, regardless of the intensity of the exercise.

The Stress Test

The first thing that is necessary before starting an exercise program is an exercise test on the treadmill or bicycle. This is very important for heart patients as it can demonstrate problems at certain pulse rates or exercise loads. For instance, the stress test can show if exercise brings on an oxygen deficit, or stimulates an abnormal rhythm, or results in a drop in blood pressure. With this information an exercise prescription can be written which would specify the amount of exercise to be utilized to start the program. A desired pulse rate and exercise time would be prescribed, but they should be reviewed routinely to increase the amount of exercise the patient can tolerate.

Question: I read recently where a man died while jogging. Is jogging or vigorous exercise dangerous?

Answer: No. With close to 3,000 men and women dying every day from heart disease, the grim reaper is obviously going to select an occasional jogger. In a large metropolitan area you could have fifty to one hundred people die every day, the majority while watching TV, washing dishes, riding on the bus, or sitting at a baseball game, but if one falls over on a high school track the story receives national coverage. These single examples are then gleefully held up as an indication that we should not use our bodies in exercise.

Exercise is anything but unhealthy. In fact, the dangers of not exercising are so severe that one famous physiologist, Par Olaf Astrand, recommends a complete physical exam to see if you can withstand the rapid deterioration of inactivity.

The actual risk of vigorous exercise is, indeed, very small. At Dr. Kenneth Cooper's Aerobic Institute in Dallas, computer information on close to 3,000 men and women taking part in vigorous exercise was analyzed. Over a five-year period this group logged 374,798 hours of exercise, which included 2,726,272 kilometers of running. The ages ranged from 17 to 73 years with an average age of 37; 1 percent had had a heart attack, 5 percent had abnormal resting electrocardiograms, and 11 percent had abnormal stress tests. There were only 2 cardiac events and no fatalities recorded. The risk was calculated at possibly 1 event per 10,000 hours of vigorous exercise but they indicated that this calculated risk was probably higher than any usual risk. When one considers that most of the exercise studies to date show decreased risks (heart attack or other problems), then the safest route to follow would be to start an exercise program immediately.

Question: I've had a heart attack and my doctor has enrolled me in a hospital exercise program where I exercise while hooked up to an EKG monitoring machine. Isn't this the safest way to go?

One would think that monitored exercise while hooked up to an EKG machine in the hospital setting is a good place to start, and indeed it is. However, both patient and physician must be careful that the patient does not develop a dependency on the hospital setting. Occasionally a cardiac rehabilitation program, with exercise always under close and monitored supervision, creates a cardiac cripple who is fearful of any activity away from the hospital. The end result of this experience is not rehabilitation but further incapacitation.

Every rehabilitation program should be geared for returning the patient to his home environment with a carefully prescribed exercise schedule to be carried out. Even though the cardiac rehabilitation programs are here to stay, I know of no studies that show that they are significantly safer than carefully prescribed programs carried out by the patient at home. An exercise program, whether initiated in the cardiac rehabilitation center or not, should have three factors:

1. It should be vigorous enough to cause an elevation in the pulse. This, as we will discuss, may be difficult with certain heart medications.
2. It should be long enough per session to be beneficial, usually thirty to forty-five minutes.
3. It should be frequent enough to be effective, and that would be at least four to six times per week.

Question: What should my exercise pulse be?

Answer: Your maximum pulse, or the pulse rate that you would achieve at maximum exercise, can be estimated by subtracting your age from 220. As we get older, our maximum pulse rate has a tendency to drop. For instance, if you are forty-five years old and are suddenly motivated to run about one-quarter of a mile being chased by a 500-pound tiger intent on making you his meal, your pulse rate would, on the average, reach about 175 (220–45).

Most exercise physiologists agree that it is not necessary to reach the maximum pulse rate to achieve good cardiovascular conditioning. Generally, exercise that sustains 75 percent of the maximum calculated pulse rate will produce beneficial effects. For our average forty-five-year-old, that would be 75 percent of 220–45, or 131. While some effects would occur at lower pulse rates, the benefits of conditioning exercise drop off sharply when the exercise elevates the pulse to less than 65 percent of the maximum calculated rate.

These numbers, using the above formula, are only an estimate. People differ markedly; certain diseases either lower or elevate the pulse rate response to exercise; numerous drugs, particularly the class of drugs called "beta blockers," alter the pulse response, and must be taken into account when starting an exercise program. While Inderal and the other beta blocker medications are quite beneficial at reducing chest pain and preventing a second heart attack, they block the normal heart response to certain hormones that would cause an increase in the heart rate. Inderal is a widely used medication, and one of the major problems I see with the use of it, and other beta blockers, is that the benefits of exercise are eliminated. If a patient is taking 120 mg (40 mg three times a day) of Inderal or more a day, he will usually have a low pulse rate in response to exercise, and will be unable to condition his heart. Inderal should be used in a rational way, by gradually decreasing it as patients improve, in order for the heart rate to respond to exercise and for the individual to achieve some benefit.

Pick a Program

Walking, walking and slow jogging, stationary bicycling, bicycling, swimming, or aerobic dancing—these are the best because you can carefully monitor yourself and follow a prescribed regimen. Racquetball, squash, or handball requires skill and a partner, and unless you're good at it, the exercise is not that great—you spend most of the time picking up the ball. Tennis, golf, and bowling simply don't count. Competitive hard singles tennis is close, but still a lot of time is spent retrieving the ball. Doubles tennis has very little aerobic conditioning power. In golf, the walking is not constant and most players ride. Bowling doesn't condition the heart. I certainly have nothing against these sports—I play them all—but they don't condition the heart and should be done for fun, only. If you count them as exercise, you may count yourself out of a more vigorous exercise program and thus miss the benefits.

Choose a Program of Exercise from these:

Walking, Walking and Slow Jogging

Advantages:

1. By far the most convenient form of exercise.
   a) Can be done anywhere at any time.
   b) More people use this form of exercise than any other.
   c) Can easily be done alone or in a group.
   d) Requires no athletic skill or talent.
   e) Most convenient form of exercise while traveling.
2. Uses the largest muscle groups, stimulating marked cardiovascular conditioning.
3. Easiest to monitor with respect to pulse rates, time, and distance.
4. By far the least expensive. All you need is a good pair of shoes which you would need for all other forms of exercise as well.

Disadvantages:

1. Slight chance of injury: foot, ankle, and knee problems can develop. Jogging does jar the system.
2. Tends to be boring unless you're really "into it."
3. Lends itself to quick and easy rationalizations—"It's too cold," "I'll walk twice the distance tomorrow," "I'm just too busy," "I just don't have time."
4. Is somewhat weather dependent. Some days it's just too cold or rainy to get out.

Bicycling at Home—Stationary Bicycle

Advantages:

1. All-weather exercise.
2. Completely safe—no jarring or weight stress on the leg experienced.
3. Can be easy to work into a routine; for instance, exercise every day while watching a certain TV show.
4. Very easy to monitor pulse and increase workloads gradually.

Disadvantages:

1. Cost. Bikes suitable for this usually start at $250 and can go as high as $700.

2. Must be done alone most of the time.
3. Can be boring.
4. Can't be done while traveling.

Bicycling on the Road

Advantages:

1. You get somewhere, covers a lot of distance—less boring than jogging.
2. Can be used as transportation to and from work if appropriate.
3. Can be done in groups—very social.
4. Can be done with the whole family—most of the time—regardless of age.
5. Can build a life-style around it, take trips, get "into it."

Disadvantages:

1. Cost. Good outdoor bicycles range from $150 or $400.
2. Dangerous; less traumatic on the legs than jogging, but one spill on a highway can be disastrous.
3. Particularly vulnerable to weather—cannot be done in cold, snowy climates.
4. Oftentimes is relegated to congested streets with auto fumes and pollution.
5. Not as "aerobic" as jogging, but certainly aerobic enough for excellent physical conditioning and providing all the benefits described for exercise.

Swimming

Advantages:

1. Very convenient, if you have a pool.
2. Can be done in warm rain (don't have to worry about getting wet).
3. Is very aerobic—uses all of the muscles.
4. Untraumatic—all weight-bearing stress is removed.
5. Excellent for those with arthritis or bone problems in the legs.
6. Excellent for those who have a weight problem; good way to get started in the exercise habit. The extra weight keeps you on top of the water. Reduces the stress of extra weight.

Disadvantages:

1. Very inconvenient, if you don't have a pool.
2. Only indoor pools suitable for all-year use in cold climates.
3. Very solitary exercise. Speaking is difficult with your face in the water.
4. Particularly vulnerable to excuses—it's too cold, I don't feel well, I don't want to get my hair wet, etc.

Aerobic Dancing

(Numerous programs of exercise to music have sprung up and are available nationwide)

Advantages:

1. Without a doubt the most fun and exciting. With Donna Summer, Olivia Newton-John, or the Bee Gees blaring away, you can't stand still.
2. Very social. Men and women in large groups participate together. Can go at your own pace and not get left by the group as with running or bicycling.
3. Very aerobic. Here at the Institute, patients routinely record the highest pulse rates during our aerobic classes.
4. Attendance and regularity good. You have to schedule the class so you feel more of a commitment to attend.
5. All-weather: indoors or can be outdoors as well.
6. Requires no special skills.
7. Uses all of the muscles as well as stretching and cool-down exercises.
8. Is loaded with examples of perfect bodies for your visual enjoyment.

Disadvantages:

1. Can be very hard on tired joints. Must be careful.
2. Can be too stressful, particularly at the beginning before you learn to pace yourself.
3. Is loaded with examples of perfect figures. Therefore, if you don't have a perfect figure there will always be a few in the class just to remind you. This can be upsetting, particularly since most of us are "deformed" by the Diet Pepsi standards.

Running Shoes

By far the most important equipment for exercise is shoes. Do not go to your closet and bring out some twenty-year-old high top black tennis shoes that have stayed with you for the last three moves. Your feet deserve better. The exercise boom has produced an incredible selection of high-quality running shoes. Put on a thick pair of athletic socks and go to a store that has a complete line of running shoes and try on several brands. You'll be amazed at how they feel, cushioning your feet like a down pillow with each step. Be sure you have plenty of room for your toes, and that there are no stress points. A good pair of running shoes, which are also the best shoes for walking and aerobic dancing, will cost from $28–$60. When you consider that in one mile of walking each foot strikes the ground over 1,000 times, you will realize that you deserve all the comfort and protection you can get. The most expensive shoe is by no means the best shoe for you—what feels the most comfortable is the best guide.

How to Stick To It

Now that we all know exercise is good for us, to help us feel better, look better, live better, and even help to save our life, some of us may start an exercise program and do very well... for about three days.

Yes, exercise is difficult, no question about it. All creatures—dogs, cats, man, and even birds—exercise out of necessity. If a dog or a cat or a lion is fed well and is not required to run and catch his meal, he will spend the whole day lying in the sun. It is safe to say that the natural inclination of all animals, including man, is not to exert. Therefore, while we may start a program of exercise, our natural bent is toward relaxation and sedentary living—sequentially we dismantle the program in a matter of days or, at most, weeks.

What we need, then, are some guidelines for success.

1. First, like any exercise program it's best to start slowly. If, with a burst of enthusiasm you try to get "in shape" in one day,

you're going to be uncomfortable and nothing dissipates resolve like exhaustion. Increases in your exercise program should come gradually and comfortably, and you should enjoy the activity. Start the program with the idea that this will be a hobby for the rest of your life. Looking down the long road of your life ahead, you'll be less apt to rush or worry about seeing immediate results.

2. Utilize methods that will enable you to stick with your program. A devoted runner once said to me that the hardest part of running was putting on the shoes. Regardless of the benefits, our natural inclination is to not exercise. To stay regular, we almost have to trick ourself into doing what we know is good for us. Here are some proven ways to keep on track:

a) Make the exercising social. Arrange to meet with two or three people of comparable physical fitness on a regular basis. This makes you obligated to go out and exercise, and works much more successfully than your own willpower. Also, this regular social activity helps make friends . . . an added bonus!

For a period of about sixteen months, I regularly met two friends at 6:00 A.M. for a five and a half–mile run. Many was the morning I would have stayed in bed if I had no commitment to meet my friends (who admitted this same fact). This regularity (four to six days a week) mounted up, and when I moved out of the neighborhood they gave me a going-away T-shirt which I wear with pride. Inscribed on the shirt is:

I RAN 1645.5 MILES
WITH TIP AND MIKE

Had it not been for Tip and Mike, I would have slept away at least half of that exercise.

b) Join a class or an exercise club. The aerobics classes are great because they are scheduled at specific times. You have already "worked it in" when you sign up. Generally if you join a group, particularly if you pay for it, you are likely to attend. As you get in condition and start feeling better, you'll begin to look forward to the music, the jumping around, and your new set of active and energetic friends. Soon the class is a regular part of your life, and you're on your way to reaping the benefits of the exercise.

c) Make exercise a part of your commute. If you can walk or ride a bike to work (and freshen up when you arrive), do it! This, without question, is the best way to be regular because you get your exercise going to work and then home—or you don't get to either place. Once I had a program where I drove my car with bicycle on the rack for 5 miles of a 15-mile commute. I then parked the car, jumped on my bike, and pedaled the remaining 10 miles. At the end of the day it was 10 miles back to the car, or I didn't get home! This, by the way, could add up in substantial savings on gas. The "gas mileage" of a bicycle, computed as calories of energy, is about 912 miles to the gallon!

But whatever exercise you choose, the important thing is staying with it. I've seen hundreds of patients blossom here at the Institute with the group walks and the scheduled aerobic classes, only to fade when they get home. Regularity is absolutely essential, and the only way to stay regular is to have built the exercise time into your day with a commitment to something stronger than just good intentions. If you start a program and falter then the structure of the commitment was not right. Don't feel bad . . . just find some formula that keeps you regular!

The Exercise Prescription

Like anything that is prescribed, the exercise prescription is unique to you. It includes:

1. a type of exercise (usually your choice)
2. an exercise pulse rate
3. frequency (times per week)
   and
4. duration

Also, the prescribed exercise program should have a gradual increase in activity that is consistent with your abilities. The best, if not the only, way to prescribe exercise is based on the results of an exercise stress test. However, the general principles are the same:

A. Type of Exercise—Must be aerobic, as discussed previously.
B. Exercise Pulse Rate—220 minus your age. The exercise or training pulse should be 75 to 85 percent of the maximum. Example:

If you are 50 years old, 220 − 50 = 170; 75 to 85 percent of 170 = a 128 to 145 range. Therefore, when you exercise, your pulse should get up to 128 to 145 beats per minute and be sustained there while exercising.

C. Frequency—Generally, exercise should be done at least four times weekly and at most six times weekly. One day of "rest."

D. Duration—One should start slow and build up to about forty-five minutes a day, divided if necessary. A typical prescription for someone sixty years old might be:

TYPE OF EXERCISE: Walking briskly
FREQUENCY: 6 times weekly
EXERCISE PULSE RATE: 220 − 60 = 160 × .75 = 120
(For the first week, do not exceed 110; build up to 120 the second week)
DURATION: 15 minutes per session for 1st week
20 minutes per session for 2nd week
25 minutes per session for 3rd week
35 minutes per session for 4th week
45 minutes per session for 5th week and then indefinitely

Record pulse reading and report any symptoms or complications at each exercise session.

PART III

The Diet: Menus and Recipes

15

General Principles of Diet

The epidemic of health problems—heart disease, diabetes, high blood pressure, even cancer—is caused primarily by our high-fat, high-cholesterol, high-salt foods. Of the commonly eaten American foods about 20 to 25 percent have no business being on your table (much less in your stomach). For many of these foods there are no substitutes, and they must be eliminated. These include egg yolks, either eaten directly in eggs, soufflés, and omelets, or indirectly as an ingredient of baked goods; most cheeses; whole milk; fatty meats; high-fat condiments like mayonnaise and most salad dressings; and, for the most part, butter and margarine. Happily, however, there is an abundance of food that *does* have a place on your table. Foods conducive to health are found in the great variety of vegetables, fruits, beans, grains, nuts, seeds, and nonfat dairy products. Utilizing these foods would help you to greatly reduce your intake of fat, cholesterol, and salt, and increase your intake of fiber. A further measure to take when using the proper foods is to learn to calculate the amount of fat they contain. Even when eating the healthful foods mentioned above, you would want to maintain an intake of no greater than 15 percent total calories in fat. This means that while some of your vegetable foods contain fat, if used sparingly, you can still keep your fat intake low in terms of overall percentage of fat calories.

Calculating the Fat Content of Foods

Most food labels contain the calories in a serving and the grams of carbohydrates, fat, and protein. In order to calculate the percentage of the calories provided by fat, you must first convert the weight of fat in grams that is present in the serving to calories of fat.

The conversion factor is 9—which means that 1 gram of fat equals 9 calories. In other words 5 grams of fat in a serving would equal 45 calories.

As far as percentage is concerned, fat is the only nutrient that you will need to monitor constantly. However, you should know how to calculate the percentage of the calories that come from carbohydrates and proteins as well. Both carbohydrates and proteins have the same conversion factor of 4. That means that there are 4 calories in each gram of carbohydrate, and 4 calories in each gram of protein.

Obviously fat is much more calorically dense than either carbohydrates or protein. One gram of fat contains 225 percent more calories per gram than either carbohydrates or proteins. That is the major reason we are so fat as a nation. By generously using butter or sour cream on our very healthful low-calorie baked potato (only 80 calories) we convert it to a high-calorie, high-fat 350-calorie disaster.

Of course, fats are necessary in human nutrition. Nature put them in foods for good reason. They contain certain essential fatty acids and are necessary in the utilization of fat-soluble vitamins, and there are other reasons, some of which we may not have yet discovered. But where we make our mistake is in consuming great quantities of fat. The typical American averages about 40 percent of his calories in fat when we need a mere 10 percent—perhaps even less. This 10 percent fat can be obtained without adding fat to our food in the form of oils, butter, or obviously fatty food. All the fat our body requires can be easily obtained from the fat in whole grains, seeds, vegetables, and beans.

For the person who needs to take therapeutic measures because of angina, previous heart attack, or diabetes, the problem of excessive fat intake becomes crucial. Fat consumption must be reduced, and a regime including high-fiber, no-salt, high-nutrient foods must be adhered to. Such a person is not a member of the preventive measures group and cannot afford to approach the program

FATS, CHOLESTEROL, AND FIBER IN FOODS

To Be Avoided[1] **high in fats, mostly saturated, high cholesterol, no fiber**	**Approx % Cal/Fat**	**Sparingly Eaten** **high to moderate in overall fats, low cholesterol**	**Approx % Cal/Fat**	**Abundantly Eaten** **low in overall fats, no cholesterol, high in fiber**	**Approx % Cal/Fat**
baked goods with egg (may have a little fiber)	45	baked goods with vegetable oils	20	beans	<20
beef	40–50	coconut[2]	85	chestnuts	<20
butter	100	fish, some	25	chickpeas	<20
egg yolks	79	low-fat dairy[3]	15	fruit, all except coconut	<20
		nuts[4]	77	grains	<20
ice cream	64	seeds	71	pasta (no-egg)	<20
lamb	34–79	soybeans	37	vegetables	<20
liver	25	vegetable oils[5]	100		
pork	43–82	wheat germ	25		
poultry	23–44				
processed meats	58–83				
veal	46–63				
whole milk	55				
whole-milk cheese	65–72				

[1]All animal foods contain cholesterol and are to be substantially reduced on this therapeutic regime.

[2]While coconut contains no cholesterol, it has cholesterol-raising properties and is categorized as a saturated fat. It is not allowed on this regime.

[3]This includes uncreamed cottage cheese, hoop cheese, farmer cheese, nonfat milk, and other nonfat (skim) milk products if available. Low-fat cottage cheese, for example, contains 12% cal./fat if 1% by weight. However, low-fat milk is not so low in fat. It is 2% by weight, or 33% by calories.

[4]While nuts are generally high in fats, they contain no cholesterol, a high level of polyunsaturated fats (only cashews and coconuts are higher in saturated than unsaturated fats), and fiber. Nuts can be used very sparingly.

[5]Oils highest in polyunsaturated fats are oils with cholesterol-lowering properties, such as safflower, sunflower, and corn oil. Other oils such as coconut, palm kernel, and palm, which is common in commercial baked goods, contain a higher level of saturated fats and cholesterol-raising properties. It is best to use the whole seeds and grains from which oils are taken instead of using the oil in concentrated form.

halfheartedly. Total recovery is best and most quickly accomplished when animal products are used as little as possible.

The table on page 179 shows some of the more common types of foods to be avoided and the types that are recommended. Those to be avoided are high in fats and cholesterol. While fats and cholesterol are not the only factors involved in disease, it has been proved that saturated fat and cholesterol in our diet do increase our blood cholesterol, and elevated blood cholesterol increases the rate of plaque formation in the arteries. The more plaque formation, the greater our risk of heart disease, among other things.

16

How to Approach the Program

At first glance this program may look impossible. The diet looks Spartan, and you can't imagine ever liking what you have to eat or getting along without your favorite foods. This first reaction is normal when starting most new dietary programs. As you learn more and get more experience and your body adjusts to the changes, it becomes easier until finally you not only like the food, but you really don't miss the foods that you left behind. You develop an acute awareness that simply to flow with the current of dietary practices in this country is dangerous.

I don't want to underestimate the effort that will be required in going on this program. It's not easy. However, it is not suggested you approach the program with the idea of easing into it. This may only prolong any discomforts. A total commitment is best.

Those who will successfully implement this program generally go through three phases.

The first phase is a general negativity, and a feeling that it is impossible to make these changes. The food, at least on paper, appears strange and unappetizing. Part of the program is that you've never considered using these foods as a major source of your calories, or as an entrée to a meal. Once you get into it, you'll realize that using beans, mushrooms, and other substitutes for meat works very well. Moreover, with some practice you can learn to like them even more! In a very real sense initial negativity stems primarily from lack of experience in either preparing or eating these foods.

The second phase is one of learning and development along with a definite improvement in your general health. Like everything in life, the task of carrying out this program lessens considerably with experience. What were once strange and weird dishes now become familiar, shopping is easier, and the uncomfortable disruption of previous routines is replaced by the pleasure of instituting new ones. During this time you will invariably notice physical improvements. You will most likely have more energy, you will be taking less medication, your blood pressure almost routinely will drop, and you will have a greater sense of well-being.

Finally, in the third phase this new program becomes no longer new. Your taste buds have changed, and you are now enjoying foods that were once foreign. Being human, you will get off track on occasion, and when you do, it is often a reminder of how far you have come. For instance, after several weeks on this program the salt on the popcorn that is generally served in movie theaters will just about knock your head off. You will wonder how you tolerated such an enormous amount of salt in the past. You'll know you have arrived when the diet is no longer a diet, but simply the way you eat, a wonderful way to create and maintain health.

Out of the thousands of patients who have completed the program at the Institute, those who enjoy the most success do not look upon this program as one of deprivation, but rather as an opportunity to improve their health and enhance their lives. Their continuing good health has become a hobby, an avocation, a labor of love. Many people begin to treat themselves almost as well as they treat their cars, and enjoy doing it.

If we say this program is easy, it wouldn't be the truth. If it was easy, it wouldn't be any good. But the benefits far outweigh the frustrations. That I know.

Priorities

When the doctor says you need
More greens, while golfing is fine,
That's not what he means.

There will be many times in your life when, while attempting to adhere to your dietary regime, you will be confronted either with temptation or the necessity of choosing the lesser of two evils. Consider all of the picnics, wedding receptions, office parties, birthday parties, potluck suppers, and family gatherings in your future. Life is built around socializing, and socializing is built around eating—at least this seems to be the case in most societies in the world.

When you are unable to obtain your ideal foods, you can learn to choose the next best thing by knowing a hierarchy of priorities, that is, which foods to choose over which.

In each category listed below the foods at the top of the list are ideal; they are lowest in fat, sugar, and salt, and highest in fiber and overall good nutrition. The foods of lesser preference are listed in descending order, with the last item in each category the least desirable.

Animal products
nonfat dairy products
egg whites
low-fat dairy products

Fruits
fresh
frozen, unsweetened
dried
canned in their own juice
canned, lightly sweetened
canned, artificially sweetened

Grains
whole grains and products (cereals, pasta, etc.)
whole grains in baked goods without added egg, vegetable oils, or animal fats
whole grains in baked goods without added egg, butter, or lard
refined grains in baked goods (white flour) without added egg or fats

Nuts and seeds
fresh, raw, unsalted (used sparingly)
raw butters, unsalted (used sparingly)
roasted, unsalted

Vegetables
fresh, raw, or steamed, plain

frozen, unsalted
frozen, salted
canned, plain
frozen, with sauces

Eating Out

Most people approach a diet regime of this nature as the end of their social life. "No more dining in restaurants," they say with a pitiful look of doom on their faces. But this just isn't so. There are, for example, restaurants coast-to-coast that feature salad bars. These all-you-can-eat delights came into vogue about the same time as the emphasis on low-fat, nonfat dairy products, whole-grain cereals, and health stores in every mall. Pizza parlors, steak houses, and hamburger chains are all realizing the people's demand for a choice, so that salad bars are becoming more and more prevalent.

When in a restaurant without a salad bar, scan the menu. You can probably order à la carte. Select a green salad with vinegar for dressing, and ask to have beets, green beans, carrots, garbanzos, onions, or any other vegetables in the kitchen put on the salad. Tell them you are almost a vegetarian and to not be stingy—pile the plate high! With the salad, order a plain baked potato and/or bread. The best bread is sourdough (not French), the second best being whole wheat or rye. White bread is the least acceptable, but it is better than giving in to meat or eggs or some other unacceptable food. Casseroles, soups, and the like are usually laden with oils, cheeses, meat, or salt. When the menu lists salads, baked or boiled potatoes, and other vegetables, choose these. Overcome your shyness in restaurants and order the quantity you desire. You may be hungry enough to eat three baked potatoes, a large plate of salad, and a basket of sourdough bread. Don't hesitate to ask for seconds.

Beverages to select when dining away from home can include water, club soda, Perrier with a twist of lemon or lime, unsweetened fruit juices (particularly orange, prune, and apple), or nonfat milk. In the hot-beverage category it is easy to carry herb tea bags or grain beverages along when you travel or are invited out. Simply ask the waitress or hostess for a cup of hot water. Beverages are a necessity when consuming a large quantity of salt, but perhaps you will find that on your new diet you aren't so thirsty.

When you encounter a situation where you have no say in the menu, choose those foods closest to your ideal diet. (See lists in the section on priorities, page 183.) Sometimes this may mean several plates full of head lettuce with a wedge or two of tomato, but don't despair. It isn't your last meal. You'll survive until you get home where you can gorge yourself on favorite foods prepared from the recipes in this book or from comparable recipes. Otherwise, for the angina sufferer, diabetic, previous heart attack victim, or potential heart disease victim, a meal of fried chicken with gravy, three-bean salad with oil dressing, potato salad with mayonnaise, fruit salad with whipped cream, and white cake with powdered sugar frosting (a very likely meal at a wedding reception) may very well be your last.

Another situation that makes it necessary to eat away from home is when you're traveling. This is when your market is your home away from home. It can be just as enjoyable (and much less expensive) to stop at a grocery store and purchase your meals there. A few suggestions include whole-grain bread accompanied by fresh fruit; frozen vegetables cooked on a hot plate; or nonfat plain yogurt with a can of unsweetened pineapple.

Substitutions

The following is a fairly comprehensive listing of substitutes that will allow you to adapt most recipes to your new dietary program. This list is not conclusive because new products come out daily as an awareness about low-fat products grows. Low-fat dairy products are a good example.

Some foods, however, will have to be eliminated entirely if there is no substitute; but your taste buds will change, and soon you will no longer feel the need for a one-to-one substitute and can turn to a replacement instead. A sweet, juicy apple can satisfy your craving for dessert once you have reeducated your taste buds. Your enjoyment of a healthful diet can be as pleasurable as ever.

SUBSTITUTIONS

When the recipe calls for:	Use instead:	Recipes and guidelines
bacon	Bakon seasoning (for the flavor)	Available at your health food store or from Bakon-Yeast Inc., P.O. Box 19203, Portland, Oregon 97219.
bread	whole grain	See suggestions in shopping guide for market and health food store.
butter	Butter Buds	Available at your market. Comes dry in packets. Mix with water. Use in baked goods, over vegetables, or anywhere liquid butter is appropriate or use dry.
	ground sesame seeds	Use in baked goods instead of butter. Grind to a paste or "flour." Measure as you would butter.
buttermilk	nonfat yogurt/nonfat milk	Mix 3 parts milk with 1 part yogurt.
cheese (used only as flavoring in dishes, not as a primary food source)	hoop cheese or farmer cheese	Use in place of cream cheese and similar cheeses.
	uncreamed cottage cheese	Use in place of cottage cheese, cream cheese, and similar cheeses.

	sapsago cheese	Use in place of Parmesan cheese or hard cheeses that are used as toppings. Use lesser amounts where hard cheeses, baked in, are used. Use in place of blue cheese.
chocolate	carob powder	Use like semisweet chocolate.
coffee	grain beverage coffee substitute	directions on the jar or can
cottage cheese	uncreamed cottage cheese	Add nonfat yogurt to make into desired consistency or use dry in recipe.
cream	nonfat yogurt/nonfat milk	Add nonfat milk to make the yogurt the desired consistency.
cream cheese	hoop cheese or farmer cheese	Use as equals in recipes.
egg	egg whites	Use 2 egg whites where 1 egg is called for.
egg (baking)	low-fat egg substitute (usually comes as a powder)	directions on the package
	tapioca	Use 1 T. tapioca per egg. Good in pancakes, cookies, and similar foods.

When the recipe calls for:	Use instead:	Recipes and guidelines
flour	whole-grain flours	Use whole-wheat flour alone or mixed with other flours in foods that need to rise (like bread); other flours appropriate in pancakes, cookies, and similar foods.
ice cream	frozen bananas, frozen fruits	Freeze peeled ripe bananas and run through juicer. Make flavors by adding other frozen fruits along with banana.
	frozen yogurt	Freeze yogurt with fruits or flavorings. Blend for creamy texture.
jelly	lightly sweetened or unsweetened jelly	Use as you would any jelly.
mayonnaise	Miracle Blend Dressing	*Rich Brown:* Blenderize until creamy smooth 2 c. pear or apple juice and 6 T. cider vinegar; 4 heaping T. vegetable seasoning; 8 heaping T. unhulled raw sesame seeds. Makes a quart jar. Keeps in refrigerator a week or more. (Optional: Add 3 to 4 T. food yeast.) *White:* Blend until creamy smooth 1/2 c. nonfat milk (liquid); 3 T. whey powder; 8 T. hulled raw sesame seeds; 1 T. natural mustard; 1 T. cider vinegar. Makes about one cup. Keeps about a week.

MEAT		
ground beef	precooked lentils, kidney beans, or pinto beans (try other legumes as desired)	Use in Mexican dishes, chili (with no carne), Italian sauces, with egg whites and grains to make patties, in casseroles, and in stews.
poultry	mushrooms, fresh whole	Use in pasta and noodle dishes, in chow mein, in casseroles, and with rice.
fish	low-fat* varieties acceptable used sparingly	

Note: Meat substitutes are used to replace the meat found in casseroles, sandwich fillings, and other dishes. There is no substitute for a piece of meat that would be acceptable on this program. Most imitation meat is very high in fat, salt, and other undesirables, such as artificial ingredients.

milk	nonfat	Use as equals.
nuts	Use nuts sparingly, or use water chestnuts, roasted chestnuts, or Garbanzo Nuts.	Garbanzo Nuts: Soak dried garbanzos overnight; drain; bake in hot oven on cookie sheet about 1 hr. or until crispy.
oil (in cooked and baked foods)	lecithin	For baked goods, use 1 t. in recipes calling for 1/4 c. of oil. Use more liquids to make up remainder of moisture.

*Fish lowest in fat are tile, cod, halibut, lingcod, ocean perch, rockfish, and sea bass.

When the recipe calls for:	Use instead:	Recipes and guidelines
oil (in cooked and baked foods)	Butter Buds	In baking and cooking, use equal amounts of liquid Butter Buds to oil.
	seeds, ground (sesame, sunflower in particular)	Use ground seeds in baked goods. Use cup for cup. Seeds contain much less than their concentrated oil in the bottle.
pan coating for baking or frying	Pam or other spray pan-coating	Use as directed on the can.
	liquid lecithin	Use like butter, spreading with a napkin on a warm dish. Use a very thin coating. (This is the main ingredient in spray pan-coatings.)
peanut butter	Nutty Butter	Blenderize 1 lg. ripe banana. While blender is running, add 2 T. unhulled raw sesame seeds, 6 T. food yeast flakes, 1/4 t. vanilla, and 1/8 t. cinnamon. Keep in refrigerator. *Note:* Various brands of yeast will make the butter taste different. Experiment to suit your tastes.
pie crust	Grape-Nuts cereal	Use the plain, original Grape-Nuts. Sprinkle into pie tin 1/4″ to 1/2″ thick. Moisten with fruit juice. It will "melt" into graham cracker–type crust upon baking the pie.

	natural flake cereal	Use a no-added-fat natural flaked cereal. Crush and mix with Butter Buds or liquid for bottom, add sesame seeds for topping. (Best used on cobblers and similar dishes.)
	rolled oats	Blenderize with sesame seeds or other seeds or Butter Buds. Use as a bottom—it dries out when used as a topping.
ricotta cheese	skim-milk ricotta	Look for ricotta that is made with skim milk and whey. Other ingredients are unnecessary.
salt	Salt Sub	Mix together 4 parts onion powder, 2 parts paprika, 2 parts garlic powder, and 3 parts cayenne pepper.
	powdered sea kelp	Use in your salt shaker in place of salt.
Note: In many recipes (i.e., baked goods) the practice of using salt has gotten out of hand. It is unnecessary. As a seasoning for foods, use herbs, onion, garlic, Salt Sub, or vegetable-broth seasoning.		
soy sauce	low-sodium soy sauce	There are soy sauces made that contain less sodium.
sour cream	nonfat yogurt	Use as equals.
	skim-milk ricotta, nonfat yogurt	Thin ricotta with yogurt for cooking.
stock	liquid off cooked vegetables or soup	Save liquids from cooking vegetables, soups, potatoes, etc., and use where stock is called for.

When the recipe calls for:	Use instead:	Recipes and guidelines
stock	vegetable-broth powder	Add water to vegetable-broth powder (from health food store) to make into a stock.
sugar, white	honey (Sweetens more, therefore you use less.)	Use 1/2 to 3/4 c. honey where 1 c. sugar is called for.
brown	date sugar	Use as equals. This is a dehydrated granulated date product with nothing else added.
corn syrup	frozen, thawed, concentrates of fruit juices (apple, orange, grape, etc.), unsweetened	Use as equals, cup for cup. Apple is the least distinctive and the most compatible with recipes.
Note: Sugar is overused. You will find that you can use much less than is called for and still achieve sufficient sweetness.		
sweetener	dried fruits	In lieu of a sugar substitute, try using raisins, dates, prunes, or prune juice. Dried apricots or other dried fruits can also be used whole or in part with the sugar substitute.
	real vanilla, almond, orange, lemon extracts	When a sweetener is called for in a recipe, use a sugar substitute; only use 1/2 to 1/4 as much and enhance

		with these. Use approximately 1 t. per 1 cup of sweetener.
whipped cream	"Whipped Cream"	Blenderize at med/high speed until frothy: 3/4 c. nonfat milk, 1 c. uncreamed cottage cheese, hoop cheese or farmer cheese, and 1 T. real vanilla.
Worcestershire sauce	low-sodium soy sauce with apple juice	Mix 1 bottle low-sodium soy sauce and 1 can thawed concentrate of apple juice.

Grocery Store Shopping Guide

Good news! It is possible to shop for the major part of your groceries in your local market. A varied and interesting array of foods can be purchased at any full-service grocery store. However, if you desire to try unusual foods not common to the everyday table of most Americans, then you might seek out a health food store or a farmer's market. The health food store offers many grains, seasonings, dressings, etc., that a market may not have, especially those prepared without sugar, fat, or salt. A farmer's market may carry specialty fruits and vegetables even when they are not in season. They obtain them from small-scale growers or from other states or countries.

Following is a categorized listing of foods found in your grocery store. It is always necessary to read labels. Sourdough bread is a good example. It is usually made of simply flour, water, yeast, and salt. But you might easily come across a sourdough bread that also contains such items as dough conditioners, fats, coloring, preservatives, etc. Labels are required to list the product's ingredients in order of greatest to least quantity. The first ingredient listed is the ingredient contained in the food in the most quantity, flour in bread, for instance. This is why you will usually find such things as salt, colorings, or preservatives toward the end of the list. Labels are meant to be read.

Beans and Grains
brown rice
split peas (yellow and green)
lentils
barley
beans (white, red, navy, pink, black, blackeye peas, pinto)
chickpeas (garbanzos)
corn meal
whole-wheat flour

Breads
sourdough
whole wheat
rye

pita
tortillas (corn)
rye crisps
flat breads
"Bible" bread (unleavened)
(Look for breads that are whole grain and have no added fat. Sourdough is not truly a whole-grain bread. It is made from white flour, but it is generally made without added fats, sugars, or preservatives. It is better to occasionally eat less-than-perfect breads than to eat animal products that contain substances far more detrimental to your health.)

Cereals
puffed, plain, corn, wheat millet, rice
oatmeal
Cream of Wheat or Rice
Roman Meal
Wheatena
Shredded Wheat (regular or spoon-size)
natural flake cereals (These contain just the whole grains, yeast perhaps, malt flavoring. No fat. NutriGrain Cereals from Kellogg's.)

Dairy
egg whites (Give the yolks to your dog or cat.)
plain nonfat yogurt
nonfat milk
sapsago cheese
hoop cheese
farmer cheese
uncreamed cottage cheese

Dressings and Condiments
brown mustard (mustard seed with vinegar and seasonings)
no-oil dressing
vinegar
honey
Butter Buds
Pam (or other pan-coating spray)

Fruits

fresh, all that are in season
dried (dates, raisins, prunes, apricots, etc.)
unsweetened applesauce (bottles and cans)
canned fruits packed in their own juice or unsweetened juice
frozen fruits packed without sugar (strawberries, cherries, peaches)
juices, unsweetened (jars, canned, or frozen concentrate)

Note: Coconut milk (liquid expressed from mixture of grated coconut meat and water) is 25 percent fat, while coconut water (liquid from coconuts) is only .2 percent fat. Coconut cream (liquid expressed from grated coconut meat) is 32.2 percent fat.[1] Some juices contain coconut "juice." Look for the fat content on the label.

Also, a juice labeled *drink* indicates that it contains other ingredients. Some may not be desirable for this program.

Herbs, Spices, Flavorings, Thickeners, and Leaveners

spices (allspice, cinnamon, cloves, coriander, fenugreek, ginger, nutmeg, pepper, turmeric, vanilla bean, etc.)
herbs (aniseed, basil, bay leaves, caraway, chives, cumin, dill, fennel, garlic, marjoram, mints, mustard, parsley, rosemary, saffron, sage, tarragon, etc.)
flavorings (real vanilla, almond, orange, lemon, anise, or mint extracts)
thickeners (tapioca, arrowroot, whole-wheat flour, potato flour or starch, agar, gelatin, cornstarch)
leaveners (live yeast, dry/live yeast, baking soda, baking powder)

Nuts and Seeds

raw in shell
raw in bags, shelled
(Nuts are generally available in the health food store in greater variety and at lower cost than in the market.)

Pastas

all pastas without added egg
(The market pastas are made with white flour. Pastas available in health food stores are made with whole-wheat flour, vegetable

[1]*Composition of Foods,* Agriculture Handbook, No. 8, Table 1, #788, #792, #793. October 1975.

"flours," and a variety of grains. These would be preferable. Pastas are the basic staple found most abundantly in your health food store.)

Snack Foods and Beverages

decaf coffee or grain beverage
herb teas
popping corn (to be popped in a hot-air popper that uses no oil. Or, popcorn can be popped over an open flame using an old-fashioned wire basket popper with handle.)
sparkling cider
Perrier

Vegetables

all frozen or canned vegetables (choose those without salt or artificial ingredients added. Or rinse well.)

Let's not throw the baby out with the bath water. If you take the time and effort and loving care to wash the baby, don't throw him out with the bath water. In the same way, don't sacrifice the health of the remainder of your body in your efforts to have a healthy heart or pancreas. Saccharin, for example, is suspected of being a carcinogen, so much so, that most stores post warnings to this effect. What good is a healthy heart if you risk acquiring some other malady? Besides, who needs saccharin? There are plenty of alternative sweeteners that work, and that are allowable and health-promoting in small quantities. Instead, we can use honey, concentrated fruit juices, or flavor enhancers, like extracts or spices, that fool our taste buds. Keeping this in mind, whatever food product you buy, read the label. Avoid chemicals. Strive to purchase whole, unprocessed foods that promote total health.

Health Food Store Shopping Guide

Most health food stores carry large selections of the following items. If you can't find something, ask that it be ordered for you.

baking items (liquid lecithin, baking powder)

beans
breads, crackers (made without added fats, salt, or sugar)
canned goods (vegetables, tomato paste, fruits—all without added salt, sugar, fats)
cereals (for cooking, or ready-to-eat)
coffee substitutes (grain beverages)
condiments (mustard, catsup)
drinks (natural sodas)
dressings for salad (no-oil, either bottled or package that you mix up at home)
flavorings (natural extracts)
grains (millet, buckwheat, rye, wheat, etc.)—whole, or ground into flours
herb teas
juices (bottled or some health food stores carry fresh varieties)
nutritional foods (brewer's yeast, rice polish, bran) *Note:* Yeast varies widely in flavor. Some food yeasts are bitter, others are actually delicious.
pastas
seasonings (vegetable-broth seasonings, made without added salt, that will usually contain dried vegetables, yeast, grains, garlic, and other herbs and spices)
seeds (sesame, sunflower, flax)
substitutes (egg substitute made with low/no fat ingredients, non-glutenous flours for those with wheat allergies, low-sodium baking powder)
sweeteners (date sugar, honey)
thickening agents (agar, arrowroot, tapioca)

Definitions

Agar A mucilaginous material prepared from certain seaweeds. Used like gelatin.

Arrowroot An edible starch made from the root of a tropical American plant.

Butter Buds A brand name for a butter substitute with no cholesterol. Comes in packets to be added to water for a liquid type of butter, or used dry.

Chives A plant with grasslike, onion-flavored leaves used as seasoning. Looks like very thin green onions.

Essene Bread "Bible" bread, unleavened.

Herb An often aromatic plant used in medicine or as a seasoning.

Hoop Cheese A compressed block form of uncreamed cottage cheese.

Liquid Lecithin An emulsifying substance from soybeans.

Pam A brand name for a pan-coating spray used when baking or frying. Main ingredients are usually lecithin, a hydrogenated vegetable fat, alcohol, and a propellent.

Pita Bread Pocket bread.

Perrier Mineral water. Like carbonated water.

Sapsago Cheese A very-low-fat, gratable cheese used in place of Parmesan cheese. "Green cheese."

Spice An aromatic or pungent plant substance, as cinnamon or pepper, used for flavoring foods.

Tapioca A bready starch obtained from cassava root and used for thickening puddings, soups, etc.

Vegetable-Broth Seasoning A seasoning made from the dehydrated concentration of vegetables, grains, herbs, and spices. Look for those that contain no salt.

Kitchen Equipment

Part of being successful in your healthful cooking endeavors is having access to a kitchen equipped with certain essential items. You probably already have the usual appliances and utensils: stove, oven, refrigerator, pots and pans, knives, measuring cups and spoons, bowls, eating utensils, and storage containers. These are even found in the kitchens of bachelors and newlyweds. But what you may not own are the following, which can make your cooking speedier, more fun, and allow for greater variety.

You'll use these items daily:

blender (Osterizer or comparable brand with a powerful motor)
stainless-steel steamer for cooking vegetables
nonstick bakeware (griddle, bread pans, muffin tins, cookie sheets, and frying pan)

hand mixer
colander
vegetable scrub brush
garlic press
grater
Add these as you can.

These will make life easier and more recipes possible:
hot-air corn popper (or old-fashioned wire-mesh corn popper)
spin-dryer for lettuce, fruits, and vegetables
pressure cooker
Crock-Pot
nonstick waffle iron
yogurt maker
juicer (A Champion juicer is made to perform duties beyond juicing. It features a spout for pulp ejection instead of the more common basket catcher. The spout enables the user to make mashed, pureed, and grated foods.)
double boiler (for cereals and sauces)
Mason jars for sprouting seeds, beans, and grains
sprouting lid, cheesecloth or Fiberglas screen, and rubber bands

---

Herbs and Spices

The problem with most herb guides is that they are arranged in the wrong order. What the cook needs is an herb guide that lists each food and then lists all of the herbs that are compatible with that food. Most herb guides are reversed.

Herbs and spices have varying flavors and strengths. Many herbs and spices may be delicious in one food but perhaps not at the same time. Therefore, the cook should consult the flavor guide for herbs and spices and select those seasonings that will be synergistic. Similarly, you will seldom want only one herb or spice in a dish. Certain flavors work together to create a desired effect. Cinnamon, nutmeg, cloves, and ginger, for example, are often found together in pies, cakes, and cookies. They enhance one another as well as the flavor of the food. However, the cook needs to go through a learning period first.

When you are starting to cook with herbs and spices, use only one per dish. In this way the individual flavor can be discerned. Mixing herbs and spices that you are unfamiliar with will not teach anything about seasoning. Once you have learned their individual flavors and strengths, you can mix and match to achieve wonderful results.

For those foods not listed in this chapter you might consult a recipe to see which herbs are suggested. If a recipe for an apple dish suggests cinnamon, for example, this might indicate that cinnamon would be appropriate with apples in other recipes as well. However, for some foods there are no specific seasonings. Grains, for example, are cooked in so many ways that the seasonings that are appropriate with the grain are those that complement the particular food with which they are being cooked. (Cinnamon in a fruit bread, for instance.)

HERBS AND SPICES GUIDE

Food	**Herbs and Spices**
apples, baked	caraway seed, cinnamon, cloves
apple cake	coriander, cinnamon
apple pie	aniseed, cloves, cinnamon, coriander, nutmeg
apples, stewed	allspice, aniseed, cinnamon, cloves
bananas	cinnamon
bean dishes (with tomato)	basil, rosemary, black pepper, garlic, oregano
bean dishes (with vegetables)	basil, garlic, rosemary, pepper
beans, green	basil, dill, marjoram, mustard, nutmeg, oregano, savory, thyme
beets	allspice, bay leaf, caraway seed, cloves, ginger, mustard
biscuits	allspice, poppy seed (topping)

Food	Herbs and Spices
bread, general	aniseed (seeds), poppy seed (topping), sesame seed (topping)
bread, fruit	coriander, sesame, allspice, cinnamon, cloves, ginger, aniseed
bread, rye	caraway, cumin
breads, sweet	curry
Brussels sprouts	caraway seed, mustard, nutmeg, sage
broccoli	carraway seed, mustard, oregano, tarragon
buns	allspice
cabbage, green	caraway seed, celery seed, cumin, curry powder, fennel, mustard
cabbage, red	aniseed (plus above)
cake, plain	poppy seed, sesame seed (toppings), vanilla
cake, fruit	allspice, sesame, cinnamon, cloves, ginger, nutmeg, vanilla
carob sauce	juniper
carrots	allspice, bay leaf, cinnamon, curry powder, dill, ginger, aniseed, cumin, mint, poppy seed (topping)
carrot soup	coriander
cauliflower	cayenne, celery seed, chili powder, nutmeg, paprika, rosemary, mustard powder (for sauce), paprika (garnish)
celery	paprika (garnish for filling)
Chinese food	ginger
coleslaw	caraway seed, mustard seed

Food	Herbs and Spices
cookies	allspice, aniseed, cloves, ginger, nutmeg, cinnamon, sesame, vanilla
corn	cayenne, celery seed, chili powder, curry powder, paprika
cottage, farmer, or hoop cheese, dips or sauces with vegetables	curry, mustard powder, nutmeg, paprika, poppy seed, sesame seed
cucumbers	fennel seed
dumplings	caraway seed
egg curry	tamarind (with curry powder)
eggplant	allspice, bay leaf, chili powder, marjoram
egg-white dishes (with fruits, grains, etc.)	nutmeg, allspice, cinnamon, cream of tartar (beaten egg whites), ginger, cloves, saffron
egg-white dishes (with vegetables, grains, etc.)	curry powder, mustard powder, basil, chives, marjoram, nutmeg, paprika (garnish), pepper (black or white), poppy seed (garnish), saffron, parsley, oregano, turmeric
fish	bay leaf, saffron, dill, basil, fennel, parsley, tarragon
fruit cobbler	sesame seed (topping)
fruits, dried, mixed, and stewed	ginger, nutmeg
fruits, pickled	cloves
fruit salad	cinnamon
hoop cheese	allspice, nutmeg (in Italian dishes)
lentil soup	coriander, dill seed, basil, parsley
lima beans	nutmeg, marjoram
macaroni salad	mace

Food	Herbs and Spices
melon	ginger
mustard	Mix prepared mustard with tarragon vinegar. (*See also* vinegar.)
omelet	curry powder, chives, chili powder, basil (If tomato is included, use herbs and spices for tomato.)
onions	bay leaf, mustard, oregano, paprika, sage
parsnips	aniseed, poppy seed
peaches	cinnamon
pears, stewed	allspice, cinnamon
peas	chili powder, dill, mint, oregano, poppy seed, rosemary, sage, marjoram
pea soup	coriander
pickles	allspice, cumin, fenugreek, juniper, dill
pickling vegetables	caraway seed, cardamom, cloves, ginger, pepper (black or white)
pie, fruit	aniseed, cumin (sparingly), cinnamon, cloves, ginger, allspice, nutmeg, mace (cherry pie)
pizza	(*See* tomato.)
potatoes	caraway seed, fennel, mustard, oregano, pepper, paprika, sesame seed, poppy seed, chives
puddings, milk	cinnamon, cloves, nutmeg, allspice, ginger
puddings, sponge	ginger

Food	Herbs and Spices
rhubarb	allspice, cinnamon
rice, Indian	cardamom
rice, plain	fenugreek, saffron (changes rice color as well), basil
rice pudding	cardamom, cinnamon, cloves, allspice, nutmeg
rice, with tomato	(*See* tomato.)
salad dressings	aniseed, paprika, black pepper, parsley
salads, vegetable	anise (chopped leaves), chives, paprika, parsley, pepper
salad, Waldorf	paprika
sauce, buttery	thyme
sesame halvah	fenugreek
soufflé	chilies
soup, creamed	chilies, cinnamon, cloves, curry (as garnish)
soup, vegetable	cardamom, poppy seeds (whole as garnish), marjoram, parsley, rosemary (sparingly)
spinach	allspice, cinnamon, nutmeg, oregano, rosemary, sesame seed
squash	allspice, bay leaf, cinnamon, cloves, ginger, nutmeg, paprika
stewed fruits	cardamom
stews, vegetable	rosemary (sparingly), sage
stuffings	sage (with breads and grains), oregano (with fish)
sweet potatoes	cardamom seed, cinnamon, cloves, ginger, nutmeg, paprika

Food	Herbs and Spices
sweet-and-sour sauces	cumin
toast	cinnamon
tomatoes	basil, celery seed, chili powder, curry powder, oregano, garlic, parsley, thyme, cumin, marjoram
tomatoes, Italian and Mexican dishes with	chili powder, basil, garlic, oregano
turnips	allspice, celery seed, curry powder, dill, oregano
vegetable curries	curry powder, cinnamon, tamarind, turmeric
vegetable dishes	black pepper, basil, parsley
vegetable sauces	paprika (garnish)
vinegar	tarragon (Steep 1 T. per pint of vinegar.)
waffles	sage, cinnamon, allspice, cloves, ginger, nutmeg
"whipped cream" (See page 193)	cinnamon, vanilla

Herbs and Spices Flavor Guide

Aromatics (Enhancers of flavor; they have an elusive way of doing it, like perfume)

allspice Use sparingly. Like a mixture, though it is not, of cinnamon, nutmeg, and cloves.

aniseed Use sparingly. (*See also* fennel.) Tastes licoricelike.

cardamom Use sparingly. Tastes like a ginger-cinnamon combination.

chervil Use sparingly. Has a delicate, anise-like taste when fresh. Excellent in salads, egg dishes, and with carrots.

cinnamon (cassia)	Use sparingly to moderately. Gentle, musky flavor. Enhances sweets.
cloves	Use sparingly. Sweeter than nutmeg. Woody, dark, musty flavor. Widely used.
dill	Use sparingly (i.e., $^1/_4$ t. per six servings). Of the parsley family. Sweetly aromatic.
fennel	Use sparingly to moderately. Tastes licoricelike.
fenugreek	Use sparingly. Tastes bitter.
garlic	Use sparingly. Use by the clove, which can be removed from the cooked dish. Tastes like "enriched onion."
mace	Use sparingly. Tastes like nutmeg, but more pungent.
nutmeg	Use sparingly. Cousin to mace. Woody, rich flavor. Good for flavoring green beans.
parsley	Use moderately to heavily. The common American variety has a woody flavor. Chinese variety (cilantro) is used in Latin American and Chinese dishes.
rosemary	Use sparingly. Of the mint family. Has an "evergreen" flavor.
sage	Use very sparingly. Has an earthy, musty flavor.
savory	Use moderately. The bean herb. Very mild. Similar to thyme, only milder. Lemon-mint cross in flavor.
tarragon	Use sparingly. Has a distinctive, slightly licorice flavor.
thyme	Use sparingly to moderately. Mild, fragrant taste. Very widely used.

Sweet and Bittersweet

Basil	Use moderately. Savory, vegetable-sweet.
bay leaf	Use sparingly (i.e., one leaf for six people). Bittersweet. From the laurel tree. Remove before serving the dish.
coriander	Use sparingly. Tastes like a lemon peel–and–sage combination. Bittersweet.
juniper	Use sparingly. Pinelike flavor. Bittersweet.
oregano	Use sparingly. The pizza herb. Savory, has lingering flavor. Bittersweet.
poppy seeds	Use moderately. Little flavor. Nutlike texture.
marjoram	Use sparingly. Cousin to oregano, but sweeter, more delicate. Bittersweet. One of the finest salad herbs.
paprika	Use moderately. Of the pepper family, can be mild to hot, depending upon variety. Keep jar or can tightly closed

in refrigerator. Goes stale quickly. Subtle, musty, warm taste. Sweet.

sesame seeds	Use moderately to heavily. Nutty flavor and texture.
saffron	Use very sparingly (i.e., $^1/_8$ to $^1/_4$ t. per dish). Very expensive. Mild, slightly sweet flavor. Spicy.
vanilla	Use sparingly to moderately. Sweet, chocolaty flavor.

Sharp, Peppery, Hot

Caraway	Use sparingly. Deepens the taste of things. Halfway between aniseed and fennel in flavor. Mildly sharp and peppery.
cayenne	Use sparingly. Ground red pepper. Sharp and peppery.
chili powder	Use sparingly to moderately. Vary in strength. Hot, peppery.
*cumin**	Use sparingly. Cousin to caraway. Yellow color. Sharp and peppery.
curry	Use sparingly to moderately. Actually a combination, of which there are many varieties. Use $^1/_2$ to 1 t. per six servings. Hot, spicy.
ginger	Use sparingly. Hot and peppery, spicy. Used often in sweet foods.
mint	Use moderately. Highly aromatic, clean, pinelike. Sharp, peppery.
*mustard**	Use sparingly. Hot, sharp, peppery. Yellow color.
pepper	Use sparingly to moderately. White is milder, more aromatic. Hot.
*turmeric**	Use sparingly (i.e., $^1/_4$ tsp. per four servings). Yellow color. Sharp, peppery.

Note: Sparingly means approximately 1 tsp. per four to six servings. *Moderately* means approximately 1 tsp. per two to four servings. *A pinch* means just that—a pinch between the fingers. Use approximately three times as much of a fresh herb as a dried one.

*These spices are often used solely for the color they impart to the dish.

17

Menus and Recipes

How to Use the Menu Plan

Following are twenty-one days of recipes for breakfast, lunch, or dinner main dishes, lunch or dinner side dishes, salads, breads, desserts, beverages, and brown bag meals. They are listed simply by number, so instead of using menus planned by someone else, you can choose your own daily menu according to what you have on hand, what you can afford, and what you can shop for easily. Less work, less worry, less waste.

It isn't too realistic to plan a week of menus with different foods at every meal. Most of us have leftovers to contend with and can't afford to waste them. However, for those cooks who prefer to see a menu laid out for them on paper, we've included one week of menus. This will give you an idea of how to plan, will save time, and will let you get a head start. Once you've got the idea, you can plan from day to day or by the week or month using the recipes that follow, or using other recipes with substitutes.

If you use these recipes, you can plan carefully so that you utilize the minimum varieties of foods—oatmeal can be planned for breakfast, then used in a bread, then in cookies, for example—or you can plan by closing your eyes and pointing. Or you can plan by the numbers, selecting all 19's for one day, for example. Any method you choose will work.

One-Week Meal Plan

With Calories Calculated at Approximately 1,600 per Day
(calories rounded to the nearest 5)
(Increase or decrease quantities according to individual caloric needs.)

ONE WEEK OF MENUS

	Breakfast	Lunch	Dinner
M	Oatmeal with Raisins (10—B'fasts) Nonfat milk Cantaloupe	BLT Sandwich (1—Brown Bag) Potato Salad (2—Salads) Apple	Eggplant Delicioso (1—L & D Main Dishes) Green Beans (3—L & D Side Dishes) Spinach-Mushroom Salad (10—Salads) Carob-Mint Mousse (1—Desserts)
T	Puffed Wheat with Honey (3—B'fasts) Orange Juice Banana	Egg-White Salad Sandwich (2—Brown Bag) Carrot & Raisin Salad (3—Salads) Grape Juice	Rice Dinner Vegetariana (4—L & D Main Dishes) Cucumber Slices (9—Salads) Baked Apple (2—Desserts)
W	Seven-Grain Cereal with Prunes (12—B'fasts) Apple Juice Fresh Pear	Pita Sandwich (3—Brown Bag) Fruit Salad (7—Salads) Sesame Balls (16—Desserts)	Chow Mein (7—L & D Main Dishes) Fruit Jello (5—Salads) Banana Bread (14—Breads) Berry Pie (8—Desserts)
Th	French Toast with Jelly (20—B'fasts) Nonfat Milk	Lentil-Spread Sandwich (7—Brown Bag) Banana Apple Juice	Potato Soup (9—L & D Main Dishes) Sliced Tomatoes (6—Salads) Oatmeal Bread (15—Breads)

	Unsweetened Pineapple		Fresh Fruit Ice Cream (4—Desserts)
F	Millet with Raisins (13—B'fasts) Boysenberry-Apple Juice Oatmeal Muffins (1—Breads)	Rice & Vegetables in a Thermos (10—Brown Bag) Pineapple & Carrot Salad (4—Salads) Chewy Oat-Orange Drops (12—Desserts)	Stuffed Green Peppers à la Raffaele (12—L & D Main Dishes) Breaded Mushrooms (18—L & D Side Dishes) Frozen Banana Pie (7—Desserts)
Sat	Pancakes or Waffles (21—B'fasts) Nonfat Milk Fresh Strawberries	Cream Pea Soup (5—L & D Main Dishes) Carrot-Zucchini Bread (18—Breads) Corn on the Cob	Cabbage-Bean Soup (13—L & D Main Dishes) Coleslaw (11—Salads) Bread Sticks (17—Breads)
Sun	Swiss-Style Meusli (9—B'fasts) Prune Juice Banana	Spaghetti (6—L & D Main Dishes) Basic Green Salad (1—Salads) Garlic Bread (12—Breads)	Vegetable Cutlets with Tangy Sauce (19—L & D Main Dishes) Carrots Sesame (9—L & D Side Dishes) Irish Soda Bread (19—Breads) Pumpkin Pie (10—Desserts)
	Each morning: Whole-Grain Bread Grain Beverage or Herb Tea		*Each evening:* a Beverage

	BREAKFASTS	AMOUNTS	CALORIES	TOTALS
M	Oatmeal with Raisins (10—B'fasts)	2/3 c. oatmeal	220	
	Nonfat Milk	(meas. before cooking)		
	Cantaloupe	1 1/2 oz. raisins	125	
		1 c. milk	90	
		1/2 med. cantaloupe	60	495
T	Puffed Wheat with Honey (3—B'fasts)	2 cups cereal with	110 + 45	
	Orange Juice	1/2 c. milk		
	Banana	2 T. honey	130	
		1 cup orange juice	110	
		1 lg. banana	100	495
W	Seven-Grain Cereal with Prunes (12—B'fasts)	1 c. cooked cereal with	160 + 45	
	Apple Juice	1/2 c. milk		
	Fresh Pear	1/2 c. apple juice	60	
		1 med. pear	100	
		6 med. prunes	90	455
Th	French Toast with Jelly (20—B'fasts)	1 recipe of French Toast	325 + 60	
	Nonfat Milk	with Jelly (2 T.)	90	
	Unsweetened Pineapple	1 c. nonfat milk	90	
		2 3-1/2" × 3/4" slices		
		pineapple		565

F	Millet with Raisins (13—B'fasts)	2 oz. millet	190	
	Boysenberry-Apple Juice	(meas. before cooking)		
	Oatmeal Muffins (1—Breads)	2 T. raisins	60	
		1/2 c. juice	75	
		1 muffin	85	
		(1 doz. per recipe)		410
Sat	Pancakes or Waffles (21—B'fasts)	3 (1 doz. per recipe)	300	
	Nonfat Milk	1 T. honey	65	
	Fresh Strawberries	1 cup nonfat milk	90	
		1 cup strawberries	60	515
Sun	Swiss-Style Meusli (9—B'fasts)	1/2 the recipe (using	330	
	Prune Juice	1/4 c. raisins, 1/8 c. dates,		
	Banana	& 1/8 c. almonds)		
		1/2 c. juice	100	
		1 sm. banana	80	
		1 c. nonfat milk	90	600

Each morning:
Grain Beverage or Herb Tea
without Sweetener or Milk

	LUNCHES	AMOUNTS	CALORIES	TOTALS
M	BLT Sandwich (1—Brown Bag)	2 sandwiches	300	
	Potato Salad (2—Salads)	1/2 c. salad	55	
	Apple	1 med. (2 1/2″ diam.)	60	415
T	Egg-White Salad Sandwich (2—Brown Bag)	2 sandwiches	360	
	Carrot & Raisin Salad (3—Salads)	1 c. salad	100	
	Grape Juice	1 c. juice	170	630
W	Pita Sandwich (3—Brown Bag)	2 sandwiches (using 2 T. sunflower seeds)	370	
	Fruit Salad (7—Salads)	1 c. salad	100	
	Sesame Balls (16—Desserts)	1 ball (16 balls per recipe)	70	540
Th	Lentil-Spread Sandwich (7—Brown Bag)	1 sandwich (1/2 c. spread per sandwich)	200	
	Banana	1 lg. banana	100	
	Apple Juice	1 c. juice	115	415

F	Rice & Vegetables in a Thermos (10—Brown Bag)	entire recipe	265	
	Pineapple & Carrot Salad (4—Salads)	1 c. salad with 1/2 c. dressing	170	
	Chewy Oat-Orange Drops (12—Desserts)	2 cookies (2 doz. cookies per recipe)	100	535
Sat	Cream Pea Soup (5—L & D Main Dishes)	3 c. soup	240	
	Carrot-Zucchini Bread (18—Breads)	1 slice (15 slices per loaf)	100	
	Corn on the Cob	1 ear corn	120	460
Sun	Spaghetti (6—L & D Main Dishes)	1 c. pasta with 1 c. sauce	150	
	Basic Green Salad (1—Salads)	entire recipe using 2 T. sunflower seeds	245	
	Garlic Bread (12—Breads)	1 slice (1/2″ thick)	60	455

	DINNERS	AMOUNTS	CALORIES	TOTALS	DAILY TOTALS
M	Eggplant Delicioso (1—L & D Main Dishes)	1/2 the recipe	250		
	Green Beans (3—L & D Side Dishes)	1 c. beans	35		
	Spinach-Mushroom Salad (10—Salads)	1/2 the recipe	100		
	Carob-Mint Mousse (1—Desserts)	1/2 c. mousse	332	717	1,627
T	Rice Dinner Vegetariana (4—L & D Main Dishes)	2 c. rice with vegetables	260		
	Cucumber Slices (9—Salads)	1/2 the recipe	90		
	Baked Apple (2—Desserts)	1 med. baked apple	110	460	1,585
W	Chow Mein (7—L & D Main Dishes)	1/4 the recipe	280		
	Fruit Jello (5—Salads)	1/6 the recipe	150		
	Banana Bread (14—Breads)	1 slice (10 slices per loaf)	100		
	Berry Pie (8—Desserts)	1/8 the pie	120	650	1,645
Th	Potato Soup (9—L & D Main Dishes)	entire recipe	200		
	Sliced Tomatoes (6—Salads)	1/2 the recipe	60		
	Oatmeal Bread (15—Breads)	2 slices (21 slices per loaf)	200		
	Fresh Fruit Ice Cream (4—Desserts)	1/4 the recipe	120	580	1,560

F	Stuffed Green Peppers à la Raffaele (12—L & D Main Dishes)	1 stuffed pepper	330		
	Breaded Mushrooms (18—L & D Side Dishes)	1/4 the recipe	100		
	Frozen Banana Pie (7—Desserts)	1/5 the recipe (using 1 T. honey)	250	680	1,625
Sat	Cabbage-Bean Soup (13—L & D Main Dishes)	1/4 the recipe (approx. 2 c.)	235		
	Coleslaw (11—Salads)	1/2 the recipe	250		
	Bread Sticks (17—Breads)	4 bread sticks	100	585	1,560
Sun	Vegetable Cutlets with Tangy Sauce (19—L & D Main Dishes)	1/4 the recipe with 1/4 the sauce	295		
	Carrots Sesame (9—L & D Side Dishes)	1/4 the recipe	85		
	Irish Soda Bread (19—Breads)	1 slice bread (10 slices per loaf)	85		
	Pumpkin Pie (10—Desserts)	1/8 pie (using 1/2 c. Grape-Nuts)	90	555	1,610

Each evening: a Beverage with no calories (i.e., Decaf or Perrier)

Three Weeks of Breakfast Main Dishes

Cold Cereals

1. *Puffed Millet*

2. *Puffed Corn*

3. *Puffed Wheat*

4. *Puffed Rice*

5. *Natural Flake Cereal*

6. *Shredded Wheat (Regular or Spoon-Size)*

7. *Grape-Nuts (the original, not the flakes)*

8. *Granola (made without added fats)*

9. *Swiss-style Meusli*

Per Person:

- 1 cup uncooked oatmeal (regular)
- 1 cup shredded, peeled apple
- 1/2 cup mixture of slivered almonds, raisins, dates, or dried apricots

Mix ingredients together and eat immediately. It will be chewy and dry.

Optional: Soak ingredients overnight in fresh pineapple juice or nonfat milk. Keep refrigerated.

Hot Cereals

Cook all whole-grain hot cereals in 3 parts water, 1 part cereal, using more or less water, as you desire.

10. *Oatmeal*

Variations: To cooked oatmeal, add honey and cinnamon, or prunes, bananas, raisins, almond extract (1/8 to 1/4 teaspoon), dates, or stewed apricots. The combinations are endless.

11. *Cornmeal*

Serve with honey, nonfat milk, and fruit.

12. *Seven-Grain Cereal*

Serve with honey, nonfat milk, and fruit.

13. *Millet*

Optional: Millet grain can be blenderized to a cornmeal texture. This meal may be stirred into boiling water and cooked to a porridge consistency. This will cook the millet in one quarter to one half the time it takes to cook the whole grain. Serve with honey, nonfat milk, and fruit. Raisins are especially good in millet.

14. *Buckwheat Groats (Kasha)*

Groats are pretoasted and cook quickly compared to other whole grains. Also unique to groats are their strong flavor, not too unlike slightly burned toast. Serve with nonfat yogurt and fruit or fruit juice.

15. *Wheatena*

Serve with honey, nonfat milk, and fruit.

16. *Zoom*

Serve with honey, nonfat milk, and fruit.

17. *Roman Meal*

Serve with honey, nonfat milk, and fruit.

18. *Cream of Wheat, Cream of Rice*

Serve with honey, nonfat milk, and fruit.

19. *Whole-Grain Oats, Wheat, Rye*

Whole grains require a long time to cook. Soak overnight in warm water. Cook in 3 parts water until tender. Serve with honey, nonfat milk, and fruit.

Other Breakfast Main Dishes

20. *French Toast*

Per Person:

- 2 pieces of whole-grain bread or sourdough bread
- 2 egg whites
- 1/4 cup nonfat milk
- 2 tablespoons nonfat yogurt
- 1 teaspoon cinnamon
- 1/4 teaspoon vanilla
- 1/4 cup unsweetened thawed frozen orange juice concentrate

Soak the bread in a blenderized mixture of the other ingredients. Cook on a lecithin-greased nonstick griddle, or bake in the oven on a Pam-sprayed cookie sheet or a lecithin-greased cookie sheet 10 minutes on each side. Serve hot.

Serves 1

21. *Pancakes or Waffles*

- 1/4 cup thawed fruit juice concentrate
- 1/2 teaspoon liquid lecithin
- 1 cup nonfat milk
- 1 teaspoon baking powder
- 2 cups whole-wheat flour (or 1 cup whole-wheat flour mixed with 1 cup other whole-grain flour like rice, rye, buckwheat, or oats)*
- 4 egg whites

Blenderize the fruit juice, liquid lecithin, nonfat milk, and baking soda. While the blender is still running, add the flour slowly until the mixture reaches a pancake-batter consistency. May require more or less flour than 2 cups. In another bowl beat the egg whites until fluffy. Fold the egg whites into the flour mixture. Cook on a preheated lecithin-greased nonstick griddle. Brown on both sides. Serve with thawed concentrated fruit juice or honey-packed jelly, or with pureed fresh fruits such as bananas or strawberries.
Optional: Add thawed, drained, unsweetened fruit to batter before cooking. Or use nonfat yogurt in place of the milk. Or use honey in place of the concentrated fruit juice.

*For optimum nutrition, these specialty flours may be ground fresh in your home blender.

Instant Breakfasts

When you don't have time to prepare a hot cereal and desire an alternative to cold cereal, here are three suggestions.

A. *Yeast Drink Meal*

- 1 cup fruit juice (any one you like)
- 1 ripe banana
- 1 teaspoon to 4 heaping tablespoons brewer's yeast

Optional: 1 handful of frozen fruit (blueberries, peaches, strawberries, or any kind you like)

Blenderize until smooth. Serve immediately.

Note: The varieties are many, according to the juice and fruits you choose. Also, note that the amount of yeast you use varies according to your ability to tolerate its taste. Yeasts have varying flavor; some are bitter while some are actually delicious.

Serves 2 as a snack or 1 as a meal

B. *Fruit "Smoothies"*

This is a delightful way to prepare fresh fruits quickly and smoothly turn them into a satisfying meal. The variations are endless. Use your imagination and the fruits in season for a rich supply of vitamins and raw enzymes along with nutritious yeast. Here are a few winning combinations.

#1

- Juice of 1/2 lemon
- 1 cup cubed papaya
- 1/2 cup plain nonfat yogurt
- 1 or 2 tablespoons pure maple syrup
- 1/2 cup crushed ice

Optional: 1 tablespoon brewer's yeast

Blenderize and enjoy.

Serves 2 as a snack or 1 as a meal

#2

- 1/2 cup frozen blueberries
- 1 ripe peach
- 1/2 cup filtered water
- 1 frozen ripe banana
- 1 tablespoon lecithin

Optional: 1 tablespoon brewer's yeast

Blenderize.

Serves 2 as a snack or 1 as a meal

#3

- 1 fresh mango
- 1 frozen very ripe banana
- 1 cup papaya cubes
- ½ cup apple or pineapple juice

Optional: 1 tablespoon yeast and 1 tablespoon lecithin

Blenderize and serve immediately.

Variation: Freeze your favorite juice in ice cube trays and add several to your Smoothies. This will help sweeten and chill them.

Serves 2 as a snack or 1 as a meal

C. *Whole-Grain Cereal*

- ½ cup whole grain (wheat, millet, oats, rye, rice)
- 1½ cups boiling water

Heat a thermos with some boiling water. Drain the water. Add the grain to the thermos along with the 1½ cups boiling water. Cover tightly. Do this the night before. In the morning your cereal will be cooked.

Variation: For a finer textured porridge, grind the grain in a dry blender first.

Serves 2

Three Weeks of Lunch and Dinner Main Dishes

1. *Eggplant Delicioso*

1 large eggplant
2 large tomatoes
1 tablespoon Salt Sub (see page 191)
1 teaspoon Italian seasoning (or your own mixture of equal parts basil, oregano, rosemary, and thyme)
2 teaspoons dry Butter Buds
1 tablespoon minced green pepper
4 large sliced mushrooms
4 slices whole-grain bread
sapsago cheese

Slice the eggplant into thin slices (approximately 1/4-inch thick) and lay them 1 piece thick on a Pam-sprayed nonstick cookie sheet. Blenderize the tomatoes, Salt Sub, Italian seasoning, Butter Buds, and green pepper and pour over the eggplant. Spread with mushrooms. Crumble the bread over top. Grate sapsago cheese, as desired, over all. Bake in a preheated 300° oven for 45 minutes.

Serves 4 to 6

2. *Egg White Omelet*

4 egg whites
1 cup cooked vegetables (such as cauliflower, onions, potatoes, tomato, green pepper, carrots, or broccoli)
1/4 teaspoon oregano
1 teaspoon Salt Sub (see page 191)

Beat the egg whites until fluffy. Fold in the vegetables and add the seasonings. Cook on preheated Pam-sprayed nonstick griddle until the omelet can be lifted with a spatula. Lift and turn to brown both sides.

Variation: For a zippier taste, add 2 tablespoons of Salsa (see page 239) in place of the tomato.

Serves 2

3. *Italian Dish with Broccoli*

- 4 ounces linguine, measured before cooking
- 1 cup cooked broccoli, zucchini, mushrooms, and onion
- 1/8 teaspoon basil
- 1/8 teaspoon oregano
- 1/2 teaspoon Salt Sub (see page 191)
- 6 halved cherry tomatoes
- sapsago cheese

Cook the linguine according to the package directions. Add the vegetables. Add the seasonings. Stir in the tomatoes. Pour into a Pam-sprayed nonstick baking dish. Grate cheese over the top. Cover and bake in a preheated 300° oven for about 15 minutes just to mix the flavors and heat through.

Serves 2

4. *Rice Dinner Vegetariana*

- 1 cup brown rice (long, medium, or short grain)
- 1 cup sliced carrots
- 2 cups lima beans
- 1 cup peas
- 1/2 cup sliced mushrooms
- 1 teaspoon curry powder
- 1/2 cup cauliflower florets
- 1 cup fresh broccoli pieces
- 2 teaspoons Salt Sub (see page 191)

Cook the rice according to the package directions. Steam the vegetables in another pan. Add to the rice. Add the Salt Sub and combine. Serve immediately.

Variation: Barley can be substituted for rice.

Serves 4

5. Cream Soups

Basic

- 6 medium chopped carrots
- 2 medium chopped onions
- 1 small chopped bell pepper
- 3 chopped zucchini
- 3 stalks chopped celery
- 2 large chopped tomatoes
- 1 cup chopped parsley
- 1 cup nonfat milk

Simmer all vegetables in the milk until the carrots are tender. Drain off the liquid and blenderize the vegetables until creamy, adding the liquid as needed to blend. Add 1 cup milk before cooking to serve.

Serves 4 to 6

Spinach

- 2 cups basic cream soup
- 1 package thawed frozen spinach or 1 pound chopped fresh spinach, cleaned and stemmed
- 1/2 tablespoon pepper
- 1/2 tablespoon nutmeg
- 1/4 tablespoon allspice
- 1/4 teaspoon marjoram
- 1/4 teaspoon thyme
- 1/8 cup lemon juice

Mix the ingredients well and bring to boil slowly. Remove from heat immediately.

Serves 4 to 6

Carrot

- 2 cups basic cream soup
- 3/4 cup grated carrot
- 1/3 cup lemon juice
- 1/4 teaspoon tarragon
- 1/4 teaspoon pepper
- 1 tablespoon plain low-fat yogurt

Combine all ingredients and bring to a boil slowly. Remove from heat. Serve with a tablespoon of yogurt on top of each serving.

Serves 2 to 4

Mushroom

- 2 cups basic cream soup
- 2 cups nonfat milk
- 2 cups nonfat yogurt
- 1 teaspoon pepper
- 1/2 teaspoon thyme
- 1 teaspoon onion powder
- 2 cups chopped mushrooms

Mix well and bring to a slow boil. Remove from heat and serve immediately.

Serves 2 to 4

Pea

- 1 1/2 cups basic cream soup
- 1 1/2 cups fresh or thawed frozen peas
- 1 1/2 cups nonfat milk
- 1/2 teaspoon pepper
- 1/2 teaspoon marjoram
- 1/2 teaspoon thyme
- 1/2 cup lemon juice

Mix all ingredients well and bring to a slow boil. Remove from heat immediately.

Serves 2 to 4

Tomato

- 1 cup nonfat milk
- 1 teaspoon flour
- 1 cup basic cream soup
- 1 cup unsalted tomato purée
- 1/3 cup parsley
- 1/3 teaspoon onion powder
- 1/3 teaspoon cloves
- 1/3 teaspoon pepper
- 1 tablespoon plain nonfat yogurt

Heat the milk in a saucepan. Slowly mix the flour into hot milk, stirring to keep lumps from forming. Add the remaining ingredients. Mix well. Top with 1 tablespoon yogurt.

Serves 2 to 4

6. *Italian Spaghetti Sauce*

- 1 small can tomato paste
- 4 cans water
- 4 large ripe peeled tomatoes, blended coarsely
- 3 stalks chopped celery, tops included
- 1 chopped green pepper
- 1 chopped onion
- 1/2 cup very finely chopped carrot
- 1 tablespoon basil
- 1 teaspoon oregano
- 2 tablespoons garlic powder (or 4 cloves fresh minced garlic)
- 1 cup coarsely chopped mushrooms

Simmer the ingredients for 30 minutes to an hour. Serve over any pasta.

Note: Cook the pasta in just enough water to cover. Do not drain. The pasta will retain a slippery texture similar to pastas that are served with an oily sauce.

Serves 4 to 6

Mock Meatballs

- 1 cup cooked lentils
- 1 cup cooked brown rice
- 2 egg whites
- 1/2 cup whole-wheat bread crumbs
- 1/2 cup finely chopped pecans
- 1/2 finely chopped onion
- 1 clove minced garlic
- 1/4 teaspoon oregano
- 1 teaspoon soy sauce
- 1/8 cup chopped parsley

Combine the lentils and rice with beaten egg whites. Add the remaining ingredients and form into balls. Bake on a Pam-sprayed nonstick cookie sheet in a preheated 400° oven for 20 minutes. Serve on spaghetti.

Note: Do not leave meatballs in the oven unless covered completely, as they dry out. Also, do not soak in sauce, as they disintegrate. They may, however, be served with sauce over them.

Serves 6 to 8

7. *Chow Mein*

- 1 cup snow peas
- 1 small can water chestnuts
- 8 ounces sliced fresh mushrooms
- 1 chopped carrot
- 1 tablespoon Salt Sub (see page 191)
- 2 cups defatted chicken broth
- 2 tablespoons arrowroot
- 1 package chow mein noodles

Stir-fry the snow peas, water chestnuts, mushrooms, and carrot in a Pam-sprayed pan. Simmer in water 20 minutes, or until the carrot is tender. Combine arrowroot with the chicken broth. Add to vegetables and cook until just thickened. Serve over chow mein noodles, cooked brown rice, or barley. Season at the table with low-sodium soy sauce and Salt Sub.

Serves 4

8. *Lentil Soup*

- 1½ cups water
- ½ cup dry lentils
- 1 sliced carrot
- 1 teaspoon Salt Sub (see page 191)
- ⅛ teaspoon basil
- ¼ teaspoon parsley

Simmer all the ingredients about 20 to 25 minutes, or until the lentils are tender. The water will be absorbed and the vegetables will be soupy.

Serves 2

9. *Potato Soup*

- 1 large potato (*Note:* The type of potato will affect the flavor of the soup. Any type of potato will do.)
- 1½ cups water
- ¼ teaspoon basil
- ¼ clove minced garlic
- ¼ small chopped onion
- ¼ teaspoon white pepper
- ½ cup chopped carrot and bell pepper
- poppy seeds

Cook the potato. Blenderize together with the remaining ingredients. Add the water. Simmer until tender. Garnish with poppy seeds.

Optional: Chunks of cooked potato, carrot, and bell pepper can be left in the soup, or they can be blenderized smooth.

Serves 2

10. *Millet and Brussels Sprouts Amandine*

- 4 tablespoons vegetable-broth powder
- 4 cups water
- 1½ cups millet
- ¼ cup chopped almonds
- 1 peeled, chopped tomato
- 8 precooked chopped Brussels sprouts
- 1 teaspoon almond extract

Stir vegetable-broth powder into water. Cook the millet in the water for 30 to 40 minutes. Add the almonds, tomato, Brussels sprouts, and almond extract. Simmer 15 minutes more. Be careful to watch for burning. If necessary, add more liquid.

Optional: Top with a small amount of liquid Butter Buds.

Serves 4 to 6

11. *Squash Supreme over Rice*

- 2 zucchini
- 2 yellow crookneck squash
- 1 small tomato, chopped fine
- ⅛ teaspoon basil
- 1 teaspoon Salt Sub (see page 191)
- 1 chopped scallion, white part only

Steam all ingredients together until the squash is tender. Serve hot over brown rice or barley.

Serves 2

12. *Stuffed Green Peppers à la Raffaele*

- 4 large green bell peppers
- 2 cups cooked brown rice (about 1 cup raw)
- 6 cups water
- 4 medium grated carrots
- 4 medium peeled, chopped tomatoes
- 3/4 pound chopped mushrooms
- 1/4 cup raw, unsalted, shelled sunflower seeds
- 1/2 cup chopped parsley leaves
- 4 tablespoons vegetable-broth powder (or 4 teaspoons Salt Sub) (see page 191)

Cook the bell peppers by removing the caps and seeds, turning ends up in a pot filled with 1 inch of water. Steam about 10 to 15 minutes or until tender. Stuff them with the remaining ingredients, which have been mixed together. Bake in a covered baking dish in a preheated 350° oven for 20 minutes.

Note: The peppers can be stuffed whole or halved.

Serves 4 to 8

13. *Cabbage-Bean Soup*

- 1 cup cooked navy beans
- 1/4 cup chopped onions
- 1 stalk sliced celery
- 3 diced raw potatoes
- 6 cups shredded cabbage (approximately 1 pound)
- 3 cups water
- 1/2 teaspoon crushed bay leaf
- 4 tablespoons vegetable-broth powder
- 2 cups pureed tomatoes

Combine all ingredients and simmer in covered pot for about 20 minutes or until the diced potatoes are tender.

Serves 4

14. *Minestrone Soup*

- 3/4 cup sliced carrot
- 3/4 cup sliced celery
- 3/4 cup chopped onion
- 3/4 cup green beans
- 1/2 cup whole-grain macaroni
- 1 cup sliced zucchini
- 1 quart water
- 1 1/2 cups tomato puree
- 3/4 cup cooked kidney beans
- 2 1/2 tablespoons chopped parsley
- 2 1/2 tablespoons chopped scallion
- 1 teaspoon basil
- 4 tablespoons vegetable-broth powder

Simmer all ingredients together until the carrots are tender.

Serves 4

15. *Enchiladas Ricardo*

- 1 6-ounce can tomato paste
- 4 6-ounce cans water
- 1 tablespoon Salt Sub (see page 191)
- 3 cups cooked navy, kidney, or pinto beans
- 1 cup shredded carrot
- 1 cup thawed frozen corn
- 4 ounces chopped fresh mushrooms
- 3 peeled, chopped tomatoes
- 4 tablespoons vegetable-broth powder
- 1 dozen corn tortillas
- sapsago cheese

Mix the tomato paste with 4 cans of water and the Salt Sub. Separately combine the beans, carrot, corn, mushrooms, tomatoes, and vegetable-broth powder. Dip the tortillas in the tomato paste mixture and lay flat on a Pam-sprayed nonstick cookie sheet. Fill with the bean mixture. Fold each one over and fasten with a toothpick driven in at an angle. Grate cheese over top. Bake in a preheated 500° oven for 15 minutes.

Serves 6

16. *Spanish Omelet*

- 1/4 cup unsalted tomato puree
- 1/8 cup water
- 1/4 teaspoon onion flakes
- pepper to taste
- 4 egg whites
- 4 tablespoons nonfat milk
- 1 tablespoon nonfat yogurt
- 1/8 teaspoon pepper

To make the sauce, combine the first 4 ingredients and simmer over low heat for 10 minutes. In a blender, whip together the egg whites, nonfat milk, yogurt, and pepper. Cook on a nonstick Pam-sprayed pan over medium heat until the bottom is brown and the top is set. Fill with half the sauce, and spoon the other half over the top after folding the omelet.

Serves 2

17. *Rolled Fillet of Sole #1*

- 4 6-ounce sole fillets
- lemon juice
- 1/4 teaspoon garlic powder
- 1/4 teaspoon mustard powder
- 1/4 teaspoon pepper
- 1/4 teaspoon curry powder
- 1/4 cup chopped chives
- 1 cup Mock Sour Cream (see below)

Spread both sides of the fish with lemon juice. Sprinkle both sides with garlic powder, dry mustard, pepper, and curry. Mix the chives with the Mock Sour Cream and spread one-fourth of the mixture on each fillet. Roll up the fillets and fasten each with a toothpick. Bake in a preheated 350° oven for 20 minutes or until fish is flaky.

Serves 4

Mock Sour Cream

- 1 can chilled evaporated skim milk
- 2 teaspoons lemon juice
- 3 tablespoons plain nonfat yogurt

Combine the milk with the lemon juice until the mixture thickens. Fold in the yogurt.

Makes 2 cups

Fillet of Sole #2

- 4 6-ounce sole fillets
- lemon juice
- 1 chopped onion, sautéed in water
- 3 stalks chopped celery, sautéed in water
- $1\frac{1}{2}$ cups water
- 1 cup sourdough bread crumbs or matzo meal
- 1 tablespoon parsley
- paprika

Spread both sides of the fish with lemon juice. Sprinkle the fillets with a mixture of the onion and celery. Mix the bread crumbs or matzo meal with the parsley. Crumble over the fish. Bake in a Pam-sprayed nonstick baking dish in a preheated 350° oven for 40 to 50 minutes. Garnish with paprika.

Optional: Layer another 4 slices of fish over the top of the first four slices and the topping.

Serves 4

18. *Chili*

- 1 pound kidney and/or pinto beans
- 1 finely chopped onion
- 1 stalk finely chopped celery
- 3 cloves minced garlic
- $1\frac{1}{2}$ teaspoons paprika
- $1\frac{1}{2}$ tablespoons chili powder
- $\frac{1}{2}$ teaspoon cumin
- 1 teaspoon oregano
- 2 cups peeled fresh or canned tomatoes
- 4 tablespoons tomato paste
- $\frac{1}{8}$ teaspoon Tabasco sauce
- 2 tablespoons low-sodium soy sauce or vegetable-broth powder

Cook the kidney and/or pinto beans, reserving 3/4 cup of the liquid. Simmer the beans with the liquid and the remaining ingredients in a large pot for about 1 hour. (Keep an eye on the pot for spillovers or scorching. Add more liquid if necessary.) Serve over a scoop of brown rice.

Makes 1 1/2 quarts

19. *Vegetable Cutlets with Tangy Sauce*

- 1 cup finely diced mushrooms
- 2/3 cup green beans, cut to 1/2-inch lengths
- 2 cups asparagus, cut to 1/2-inch lengths
- 1 cup finely chopped celery
- 1/4 cup thawed frozen corn
- 1 1/4 cups grated carrot
- 3/4 cup diced onion
- 1/3 cup thawed frozen peas
- 3/4 teaspoon mustard powder
- 1/4 teaspoon ginger
- 1 1/4 cup matzo meal
- 2 stiffly beaten egg whites

Steam the mushrooms, green beans, asparagus, celery, and corn about 5 to 10 minutes or until tender. In a mixing bowl, combine the steamed vegetables with the remaining ingredients, trying not to mash the vegetables. Form into patties and cover with foil. Bake on a Pam-sprayed nonstick baking sheet in a preheated 350° oven for 20 minutes. Uncover and bake to brown another 15 minutes. Serve with Tangy Sauce (see below).

Tangy Sauce

- 2 cups tomato sauce
- 4 peeled crushed tomatoes
- 1 tablespoon prepared mustard
- 1 tablespoon coriander
- 2 teaspoons Salt Sub (see page 191)
- 1/2 to 1 whole minced green chili pepper
- 1/8 teaspoon allspice

Combine all the ingredients in a saucepan and bring to a boil. Simmer for one hour. Makes about 2 cups.

Serves 6 to 8

20. *Vegeroni Casserole*

- 1½ pounds Vegeroni (whole-grain macaroni with vegetable flour added)
- 2 small chopped onions
- 3 cloves minced garlic
- ¾ cup chopped carrot
- ¾ cup chopped celery
- 1 cup chopped green pepper
- ¾ pound sliced mushrooms
- ½ teaspoon black pepper
- 5 cups tomato sauce
- ¼ cup grated sapsago cheese

Cook the macaroni and pour into a Pam-sprayed nonstick baking dish. Combine the remaining ingredients except the cheese and pour over the noodles. Grate the cheese over top. Bake, covered, in a preheated 300° oven for about 30 minutes. Bake uncovered for 10 minutes more.

Serves 6

21. *Pizza*

- 1 package live yeast
- 1 cup warm water
- 2 teaspoons baking powder
- 2 tablespoons Butter Buds liquid
- 2 tablespoons honey
- 2½ cups whole-wheat flour
- Italian Spaghetti Sauce (see page 229)
- Salt Sub (see page 191)
- chopped onion
- chopped green pepper
- mushroom slices
- grated sapsago cheese for garnish

Make the crust by dissolving the yeast in the warm water. Add the baking powder, Butter Buds liquid, and honey and work into the flour until a thick bread-dough consistency is reached. Roll the dough onto a heavily Pam-sprayed pizza pan. Let rise for 15 minutes. Flatten with your hands—thickness is a matter of preference. Bake the crust in a preheated 425° oven for about 10 minutes or until browned. Spoon spaghetti sauce onto crust and top with Salt Sub as desired, chopped vegetables, and grated cheese. Bake at 425° for 5 to 10 minutes or until done.

Makes 1 large or 2 small pizzas; serves 6 to 8

Sauces

Mushroom Gravy

- 3 tablespoons arrowroot or cornstarch, or 6 tablespoons flour
- 1 large chopped onion
- 1 pound sliced mushrooms
- 4 cups water
- 1 package no-oil salad dressing mix (preferably a garlic and cheese type)
- 2 tablespoons low-sodium soy sauce

Make a paste by stirring cold water into the thickener until a cream consistency is reached. Sauté the onion in water or a Pam-sprayed nonstick pan. Add the mushrooms. Stir until browned or beginning to cook. Cover with the water. Add the salad dressing mix and the soy sauce. When very hot, stir in the thickener. Continue to stir until smooth. Allow to boil lightly. Remove from heat and cover. Use as soon as possible. Best over baked potatoes, mashed potatoes, pasta, rice, or bread. Can also be used over vegetables.

Makes about 6 cups

Salsa

1 small can chopped sweet red bell peppers
1 large chopped onion
1 small can chopped green chili peppers
1 small can peeled tomatoes, chopped
Salt Sub (see page 191)
Tabasco sauce

Combine the first 4 ingredients. Add Salt Sub and Tabasco to taste. The amount of chili peppers and Tabasco will determine the mildness or hotness of the salsa.

Makes about 4 cups

Lemon Sauce

2 tablespoons arrowroot
1/2 teaspoon Salt Sub (see page 191) or powdered sea kelp
1 cup water
2 tablespoons food-grade linseed oil
2 tablespoons lemon juice
1 teaspoon grated lemon rind

Stir the arrowroot, Salt Sub or sea kelp, and water together in saucepan over medium heat. Stir constantly until thick. Simmer covered on low heat for 10 minutes. Remove from heat and blend in oil, lemon juice, and lemon rind. Beat well with wire whisk. Serve hot on vegetables.

Makes about 1 1/2 cups

Additional Main Dishes

Bavarian Potatoes

- 4 cups hot mashed potatoes
- 3 cups crumbled hoop cheese or farmer cheese
- 3/4 cup plain nonfat yogurt
- 1/2 finely chopped onion
- 2 1/2 teaspoons Salt Sub (see page 191) or powdered sea kelp
- Butter Buds or food-grade linseed oil
- slivered almonds
- bread crumbs
- paprika

Mix the first 5 ingredients. Pour into Pam-sprayed nonstick baking dish. Brush top with Butter Buds or linseed oil. Top with almonds and bread crumbs and sprinkle with paprika. Bake in a preheated 350° oven 30 to 40 minutes.

Serves 4 to 6

Green Rice Casserole

- 2 tablespoons food-grade linseed oil
- 1 clove minced garlic
- 1/2 cup chopped onion
- 1/2 cup chopped celery
- 1 cup pine nuts
- 1/2 cup chopped parsley
- 1 cup crumbled hoop cheese or farmer cheese
- 4 egg whites beaten frothy
- 1 teaspoon Salt Sub (see page 191)
- 2 cups nonfat milk
- 2 cups cooked brown rice

Heat skillet, add oil, and sauté garlic, onion, and celery. When almost tender, add pine nuts. Stir quickly about 1 minute. Remove from heat. Mix remaining ingredients. Add sautéed vegetables. Pour into a nonstick Pam-sprayed baking dish. Bake in a preheated 350° oven for 30 to 40 minutes or until firm.

Serves 4

Tamale Pie

Filling:

- 1 chopped onion
- 1 chopped bell pepper
- 1 stalk chopped celery
- 1 minced garlic clove
- 2 tablespoons food-grade linseed oil
- 2 cups tomato sauce
- 3 cups cooked mashed pinto beans
- 2 cups fresh or frozen corn
- 1½ teaspoons chili powder
- 1 4-ounce can sliced or chopped black olives
- 1 cup crumbled hoop cheese or tofu

Crust:

- 1 cup stone-ground cornmeal
- 1 cup cold water
- ½ teaspoon Salt Sub (see page 191)
- 2 tablespoons food-grade linseed oil
- 1 cup boiling water

Sauté onion, pepper, celery, and garlic in oil. Blend tomato sauce, pinto beans, corn, chili powder, and olives with sautéed vegetables. Pour into baking dish. Top with hoop cheese or tofu. Blend cornmeal with cold water. Add Salt Sub and linseed oil to boiling water. Now add the cold water–cornmeal mixture to the boiling-water mixture and stir until thickened. Spread cornmeal mixture evenly over casserole and bake uncovered in a preheated 350° oven for 40 to 50 minutes.

Serves 6

Noodle-Almond Casserole

- 8 ounces whole-grain pasta (wheat, spinach, corn, or artichoke)
- 1 tablespoon food-grade linseed oil

Sauce:

- 1 teaspoon vegetable-broth powder
- 2 tablespoons water
- 1/2 cup chopped onion
- 1/2 cup chopped celery
- 1 cup chopped mushrooms
- 1 cup fresh or frozen peas
- 2 cups nonfat milk
- 1 tablespoon vegetable-broth powder
- 1/4 cup whole-wheat flour
- 2 tablespoons food-grade linseed oil
- 4 ounces hoop cheese or farmer cheese
- 1/3 cup finely chopped almonds

Topping:

- 1/2 cup whole-grain bread crumbs
- 1 cup grated sapsago cheese
- 1/3 cup finely chopped almonds
- paprika
- sliced tomatoes
- fresh parsley

Drop the pasta in 3 to 4 quarts of rapidly boiling water and add 1 tablespoon linseed oil. Turn down to a low boil and cook 7 to 10 minutes or until tender. Do not overcook. Drain and set aside.

Dissolve 1 teaspoon vegetable-broth powder in water and simmer. Sauté onion, celery, mushrooms, and peas in this mixture. Add milk and 1 tablespoon vegetable-broth powder, stir, and remove from heat. Put whole-wheat flour in a small bowl and make a paste by adding 2 tablespoons linseed oil, stirring quickly so that it does not lump. Add this paste to the vegetable mixture, stirring well. Sauce will thicken gradually. Simmer 5 to 10 minutes, stirring occasionally.

Pour sauce over noodles and add hoop cheese and almonds. Mix well. Pour into a Pam-sprayed nonstick baking dish and top with bread crumbs, sapsago cheese, and almonds. Garnish with a sprinkling of paprika and bake uncovered in a preheated 350° oven for 30 to 40 minutes. Serve with sliced tomatoes and a sprig of parsley.

Serves 4 to 6

Three Weeks of Lunch and Dinner Side Dishes

Side Dishes

Choose a side dish that complements your main dish in that it is of a different color, texture, taste, and food source. If your main dish is red, choose a green side dish. If your main dish is creamy, choose a crunchy side dish. If your main dish is strongly flavored, choose a mild side dish. And if you are featuring grains in your main dish, choose a nonstarchy side dish.

1. *Steamed Artichokes*

4 large artichokes
1 bay leaf
1/2 teaspoon tarragon
1/4 teaspoon dill
1/2 cup liquid Butter Buds

Steam the artichokes in 1 inch of water that has been spiced with the herbs. Requires approximately 45 minutes to cook.

Serve with liquid Butter Buds for dipping.

Serves 4

2. *Asparagus*

6–8 stalks asparagus per person
cubed whole-wheat bread
Salt Sub (see page 191)
dry Butter Buds

Steam the asparagus for 8 to 10 minutes or just until tender. Toast the cubed bread on a Pam-sprayed nonstick cookie sheet in a preheated 400° oven after seasoning with Salt Sub (a light sprinkle over all) and the Butter Buds (also a light sprinkle over all). Crumble the bread mixture over the hot asparagus before serving.

Serves 1

3. *Green Beans*

- 1 pound green beans
- 1 teaspoon thyme
- 1 teaspoon basil
- 1 teaspoon garlic powder

Steam for 7 to 10 minutes, seasoning each of the four servings with one-fourth of the mixture of thyme, basil, and garlic powder.

Serves 4

4. *Beets*

- 1 pound beets
- $\frac{1}{4}$ teaspoon ground cloves
- $\frac{1}{4}$ teaspoon allspice
- $\frac{1}{4}$ teaspoon ginger

Steam beets whole for 20 to 30 minutes or until tender. Peel. Combine ground cloves, allspice, and ginger. Sprinkle over each serving.

Serves 4 to 6

5. *Broccoli*

Steam whole heads (cut off any large stump ends) until tender. Requires about 10 to 15 minutes.

6. *Brussels Sprouts*

Steam whole until tender. Requires about 10 to 15 minutes.

7. *Cabbage Side Dish*

- 4 cups shredded red or green cabbage
- 3 onions, chopped fine
- 2 lemons, juiced
- 4 unpeeled diced Pippin apples
- 1/4 cup apple cider
- 3 tablespoons honey
- 4 tablespoons sesame seed ground until pasty
- 1 tablespoon caraway seed
- 1/2 cup seedless raisins
- 1/8 teaspoon ground allspice

Simmer all ingredients together in a covered saucepan for about 10 minutes.

Serves 4 to 6

8. *Cabbage and Potatoes*

- 4 unpeeled diced potatoes
- 1 medium chopped onion
- 1/2 head chopped green cabbage
- 2 stalks chopped celery
- 2 sliced carrots
- 1/4 teaspoon fennel
- 1/4 teaspoon caraway seed

Steam all together in enough water to keep from burning. Steam for about 10 minutes. Add the caraway and fennel and continue cooking for 10 more minutes.

Serves 4 to 6

9. *Carrots Sesame*

- 6 scrubbed carrots
- 6 teaspoons sesame seed, hulled or unhulled
- 6 teaspoons dry Butter Buds
- fresh parsley sprigs

Steam the carrots until *al dente.* Combine the sesame seed with the Butter Buds and sprinkle over the hot carrots. Garnish with parsley.

Optional: Before garnishing the carrots, they can be baked in the oven for 10 minutes on Broil to brown. Garnish with parsley after removing from the oven.

Serves 2 or 3

10. *Cauliflower*

Steam cauliflower until tender (approximately 7 to 10 minutes). Dress with Butter Buds liquid. Garnish with poppy seed and/or paprika.

11. *Corn on the Cob*

Bring water to boil in a large pot. Drop cleaned corn into the water. Cook for 8 to 10 minutes if the corn is young and tender; 15 to 20 minutes if it is older. Serve hot. Eat plain or with Butter Buds liquid and/or Salt Sub (see page 191).

12. *Greens di Grace*

- 2–4 bunches greens (dandelion, spinach, mustard, etc.)
- water
- 1–4 peeled chopped tomatoes
- 2–4 unpeeled cubed potatoes
- Salt Sub (see page 191)

Clean and destem greens. In a large pot, put 2 inches of water and the greens. Steam until they start to wilt. Add tomatoes and potatoes—1 potato per bunch of greens. Continue cooking until the potatoes are tender. During the last 5 minutes of cooking, season with 1 teaspoon Salt Sub per bunch of greens.

Serves 1 per bunch of greens

13. *Okra*

1 pound okra
1 medium chopped onion
1 clove minced garlic
1 cup unsalted tomato juice
1 teaspoon oregano

Optional: 1/4 cup sapsago cheese

Mix everything but the bread. Place mixture in baking dish and sprinkle with bread crumbs. Bake in a preheated 350° oven for 45 minutes.

Optional: Before baking, grate cheese over top.

Serves 4

14. *Yogurt-Creamed Spinach*

1 10-ounce package thawed frozen spinach or 1 large bunch fresh
1/4 cup nonfat yogurt
1/2 teaspoon onion powder
1/4 teaspoon nutmeg

Cook spinach. Drain. Blend yogurt with onion powder and nutmeg. Stir seasoned yogurt into spinach. Serve immediately.

Serves 2 to 4

15. *Yams*

1 small yam per person

Look for yams that are deep purple or deep orange and have smooth skins. They must be hard, not soft. If the yam is particularly large, it can be halved or quartered for quicker cooking.

Gently scrub the skins with water. Place on a baking sheet. Bake in a preheated 350° oven for 1 hour if small or cut, 1 1/2 hours if larger, and 2 full hours if you have a huge yam (about 2 to 3 pounds in weight).

Allow to cool in the oven for about 1/2 hour. You can eat the yam, skin and all. No need to add anything.

16. *Potatoes*

1 russet baking potato per person

Gently scrub the potato with a brush and water. Bake in a preheated 350° oven for 1 hour. Turn the oven off and leave the potatoes in the oven, door closed, for an additional 1/2 hour. Eat, jacket and all, sandwich-fashion, or cut and fill with Mushroom Gravy (see page 238) or Salsa (see page 239) or liquid Butter Buds.

17. *Beets and Pineapple Sonia*

1 undrained can plain beet slices
1 can unsweetened pineapple chunks in their own juice
1 tablespoon arrowroot

Combine the beets and pineapple with their liquids in a saucepan. Turn on low heat. Make a paste of the arrowroot by adding water to it until a creamy consistency is reached. Stir into the simmering beets and pineapples. Cook to thicken the sauce. Serve warm.

Serves 4 to 6

18. *Breaded Mushrooms*

1 pound fresh raw mushroom caps
4 beaten egg whites
4–6 crumbled whole-grain bread slices
4 teaspoons Salt Sub (see page 191)

Dip the cleaned mushrooms into the egg whites and spread on a Pam-sprayed nonstick cookie sheet. Combine the bread crumbs with the Salt Sub and sprinkle over the mushrooms. Bake in a preheated 350° oven for 15 to 20 minutes or until tender and crisp.

Serves 6 to 8

19. *Brown Rice*

1 cup rice	$2^1/_2$ cups water

Place rice in a baking dish that has a tight-fitting lid. Cover with the water. Place in a preheated 400° oven. Cook covered for 1 hour. The rice will absorb all the water and cook to perfection. Can be seasoned with basil, saffron, garlic, onions, or pepper, separately or in combination, as desired, before cooking. Eat plain or with soy sauce.

Serves 5

20. *Mixed Vegetables*

Red, yellow, orange, white vegetables	Green vegetables

Generally mix vegetables first according to a variety of colors. But be cautious in adding more than one strong-flavored vegetable, such as cabbage, turnips, rutabagas, or Brussels sprouts, to your mixture. Steam vegetables until tender.

21. *Winter Squash*

1 acorn, butternut, or banana squash	1 tablespoon honey
4 tablespoons liquid Butter Buds	1 teaspoon nutmeg
	1 teaspoon cinnamon

Halve one squash and remove the seeds. Place in an uncovered baking dish with the insides up. Brush with a mixture of Butter Buds, honey, nutmeg, and cinnamon. Bake in a preheated 300° oven for 1 hour.

Serves 2 to 4

Additional Side Dishes

Garden-Fresh Zucchini Soup

- 3 medium zucchini
- 2/3 cup water
- 1 tablespoon vegetable-broth powder
- 2 tablespoons liquid lecithin

Chop the zucchini into 1-inch chunks and steam in the water for 3 to 4 minutes only. Do not overcook. Put in the blender with the cooking water, vegetable-broth powder, and lecithin and blenderize. Serve hot.

Serves 2

Curried Rice Salad

- 1/2 cup slivered almonds
- 2 cups chilled, cooked brown rice
- 1/4 teaspoon curry powder
- 1/2 cup Tofu Mayonnaise (see page 265)
- 1/2 cup finely chopped celery

Toast the almonds by placing them in a dry skillet over medium-high heat and shaking the pan quickly. Place all the ingredients in a chilled bowl and toss lightly. Serve at once on a bed of fresh crisp greens such as spinach, lettuce, or bean sprouts.

Serves 2 to 4

Stuffed Mushrooms

- 12 large mushrooms
- 1/2 cup food-grade linseed oil
- 1/2 cup fine whole-grain bread crumbs
- 2 tablespoons minced parsley
- 1 tablespoon minced onion

Remove the mushroom stems and set the caps aside. Chop the stems finely and place in a mixing bowl. Add the other ingredients. Stuff the caps with this mixture and broil or bake until the caps are tender.

Serves 4 to 6

Three Weeks of Salad Suggestions

1. *Basic Green Salad*

- 1 head romaine, butterleaf, redleaf, or greenleaf lettuce
- 1 grated carrot
- 1 wedge shredded cabbage
- 1 sliced large tomato
- 1/4 cup raw hulled sunflower seeds
- 2 ounces alfalfa sprouts
- 5 ounces thawed frozen peas

Wash and tear lettuce into a 6-quart bowl. Add the grated carrot, cabbage, and remainder of ingredients. Toss well with your favorite dressing from the recipes following the salad recipes or a store-bought no-oil dressing.

Serves 2 to 4

2. *Potato Salad*

- 2 cups cooked, cubed potatoes
- 1 small chopped onion
- 1/2 cup chopped celery
- 3 chopped hard-boiled egg whites
- 1 teaspoon Salt Sub (see page 191)
- 1 tablespoon vinegar
- 1 teaspoon mustard powder
- 1/2 cup plain nonfat yogurt

Combine all ingredients well. To blend flavors, refrigerate a few hours before serving.

Serves 2 to 4

3. *Carrot and Raisin Salad*

- 6 large shredded carrots
- 1/2 cup raisins
- 1 1/2 cups plain nonfat yogurt

Blend all ingredients well. To blend flavors, refrigerate a few hours before serving.

Serves 6 to 8

4. *Pineapple and Carrot Salad*

- 8 shredded carrots
- 1/2 cup crushed unsweetened pineapple fruit dressing

Mix together and serve with dressing.

Serves 4

5. *Fruit Jello*

- $1^3/_4$ cups fruit juice
- $^1/_4$ cup thawed frozen orange juice concentrate
- 1 package unflavored gelatin
- 1 large ripe banana
- $2^1/_2$ cups crushed unsweetened pineapple
- 8 ounces nonfat yogurt

Bring the fruit juice to a boil and stir in the orange juice concentrate. In a large bowl, pour the dry gelatin, adding the hot juice mixture until the gelatin is completely dissolved. Refrigerate until it is slightly thickened. Blenderize the banana, pineapple, and yogurt. Mix the gelatin mixture with the blenderized mixture until smooth or chunky, as you desire. Pour into a 2-quart mold or individual molds. Chill until set.

Serves 6 to 8

6. *Sliced Tomatoes*

- 2 large tomatoes
- 1 small Bermuda onion
- celery seed
- fresh parsley
- no-oil Italian dressing

Slice the tomatoes and onions onto individual salad plates. Sprinkle lightly with celery seed and garnish edges with parsley. Serve with Italian dressing.

Serves 4 to 6

7. *Fruit Salad*

- 1 large ripe banana
- 1 fresh papaya
- 1 large peeled, sectioned navel orange
- 1 cored, peeled, and cubed apple

Optional: seedless grapes, strawberries, peach slices, blueberries, or guava slices.

Combine fruits as desired. Refrigerate to combine flavors.

Serves 4 to 6

8. *Half Grapefruit*

Halve a grapefruit and section it by sliding a sharp knife around each section inside. Top the fruit with a spoonful of fresh blueberries or thawed, unsweetened frozen blueberries or a strawberry, or other berries. Or a dollop of nonfat yogurt can also top the grapefruit.

Serves 1

9. *Cucumber Slices*

- 1/4 cup vinegar
- 4 ounces nonfat yogurt
- 1 teaspoon dill
- 1 tablespoon apple juice concentrate (thawed)
- 1/4 teaspoon black pepper
- 1 large cucumber, peeled and sliced very thin
- 1 small thinly sliced Bermuda onion

Make a dressing of the first 5 ingredients. Marinate the cucumber-and-onion slices in the dressing overnight or all day.

Serves 4

10. *Spinach-Mushroom Salad*

- 1 large bunch spinach, washed and stemmed
- 4 ounces mushrooms, washed and sliced
- 2 chopped hard-boiled egg whites
- 1 small chopped Bermuda onion
- no-oil Italian or herb dressing

Combine first 4 ingredients and serve with dressing.

Serves 2 to 4

11. *Coleslaw*

- 1 package no-oil salad dressing mix
- ½ head shredded cabbage (or mix purple with green)
- 2 large shredded carrots
- 1 small chopped green pepper
- 2 chopped scallions
- ¼ teaspoon garlic powder
- 1 tablespoon celery seed
- 1 teaspoon mustard powder
- 1 cup plain nonfat yogurt

Prepare dressing, using the recommended amount of vinegar. Combine with other ingredients. Mix and refrigerate overnight.

Serves 4 to 6

12. *Melon Salad*

- watermelon
- honeydew
- cantaloupe
- fresh mint

Cut all melons into 1-inch chunks. Combine and serve ice-cold. Garnish each dish with a sprig of mint.

Serves 1 person per cut of melon

13. *Bean Salad*

- 1 cup cooked kidney beans
- 1 cup cooked green beans
- 1 cup cooked garbanzo beans
- 1 small chopped Bermuda onion
- 1/2 large chopped green pepper
- 1/2 large chopped red pepper
- 1/2 cup no-oil Italian dressing
- 3 tablespoons thawed frozen apple juice concentrate
- 1 teaspoon Salt Sub (see page 191)
- 1 teaspoon vegetable-broth powder

Mix the first 6 ingredients. Whisk together the Italian dressing with the last 3 ingredients. Use this to marinate the beans and other vegetables in the refrigerator overnight or all day.

Serves 6 to 8

14. *Macaroni Salad*

- 3 cups cooked whole-grain macaroni
- 1 small chopped onion
- 3 chopped hard-boiled egg whites
- 1/2 chopped red bell pepper
- 1/3 cup Miracle Blend Dressing (see page 188)

Toss together all the ingredients. Refrigerate overnight or all day to blend the flavors.

Serves 4 to 6

15. *Marinated Broccoli*

- 1/2 cup broccoli florets
- no-oil Italian or Thousand Island salad dressing

Steam broccoli florets for 5 minutes and let cool. Marinate florets for 24 hours in enough dressing to cover thoroughly. Serve with tomato slices, or with thawed frozen corn and chopped red bell pepper tossed together.

Serves 1

16. *Chinese Salad*

- 1/4 pound mung bean sprouts
- 1/2 small Bermuda onion, sliced thin
- 1 pound halved cherry tomatoes
- 1 small can chopped water chestnuts or 1/4 pound sliced jicama

Toss together all ingredients.

Serves 4

17. *Vegetables in Mustard Vinaigrette*

- 2 cups broccoli florets
- 3 sliced carrots
- 1/4 cup white wine vinegar
- 1/2 teaspoon mustard powder
- 1/4 teaspoon celery seed
- pinch of pepper
- 3/4 cup no-oil herb dressing
- 1/4 pound sliced raw mushrooms

Steam the broccoli and the carrots for 5 minutes and let cool. Mix well the vinegar, mustard, celery seed, and pepper. Beat in the herb dressing. Place vegetables in a shallow dish, add mushrooms, and cover with the dressing. Cover dish and chill 3 hours. Remove with slotted spoon. Serve over lettuce leaves.

Serves 4

18. *Peas and Mushroom Salad*

- 1 10-ounce package thawed frozen peas
- 4 ounces sliced raw mushrooms
- 1 chopped scallion
- 1/4 cup raw hulled sunflower seeds
- 1/4 chopped red bell pepper
- 1/4 cup no-oil salad dressing (your favorite)

Toss all ingredients together. Serve cold.

Serves 4

19. *Rice and Bean Salad*

- 1/2 cup cooked rice
- 1 cup cooked red kidney or pinto beans or 1 8-ounce can red kidney or pinto beans
- 2 chopped hard-boiled egg whites
- 1/2 small onion, chopped fine
- 1 tablespoon pickle relish
- 1/8 cup no-oil creamy salad dressing
- 1/8 teaspoon pepper
- 1/8 teaspoon celery seed
- 1 small head Boston lettuce

Mix all ingredients except lettuce and chill for 2 hours. Serve on lettuce.

Serves 2 to 4

20. *Dandelion Greens Salad*

- 1 4-quart bowl washed, stemmed dandelion greens
- 1/4 cup raw, hulled sunflower seeds
- 2 large chopped tomatoes
- 1 large shredded carrot
- 1/4 cup no-oil salad dressing

Toss all together.

Serves 4 to 6

21. *Apple Salad*

- 1 peeled, cored, and cubed red apple (peeling optional)
- 1 peeled, cored, and cubed green apple (peeling optional)
- Fruit Salad Dressing (see pages 260–261)
- 1 peeled, cored, and cubed yellow apple (peeling optional)
- 1/2 cup seedless raisins
- 1/4 cup chopped unblanched almonds

Combine all ingredients and serve with enough dressing to moisten thoroughly.

Serves 3 to 4

Additional Salad Recipes

Spinach Salad

- 1 pound fresh spinach
- 2 cups fresh sliced mushrooms
- 1 cup pine nuts
- 1 chopped Bermuda onion
- French dressing

Wash and stem spinach and tear into bite-size pieces. Serve on chilled salad plates and top with mushrooms and a sprinkle of pine nuts and chopped onion. Serve with a clear French dressing.

Serves 6

Carrot Sunshine Salad

- 2 cups grated raw carrot
- 1 cup fresh pineapple chunks
- 2 oranges, peeled and cut into neat sections
- 1/2 cup raisins
- 1 cup sunflower seeds
- 1/4 cup plain nonfat yogurt

Mix all together and chill for several hours before serving.

Serves 4 to 6

Salad Dressings

1. *Bottled no-oil salad dressing. Available in health food stores and markets.*

2. *Packaged no-oil salad dressings. Available in health food stores and markets.*

3. *Miracle Blend Dressing (see page 188)*

4. *Fruit Salad Dressing #1*

- 2 cups plain nonfat yogurt
- 1/2 cup drained unsweetened pineapple
- 1/2 cup unsweetened pineapple juice

Blenderize all ingredients until smooth.

Makes 3 cups

5. *Fruit Salad Dressing #2*

- 2 cups plain nonfat yogurt
- 1/2 cup any unsweetened fruit
- 1/2 cup any unsweetened fruit juice

Blenderize all ingredients until smooth.

Makes 3 cups

6. *Fruit Salad Dressing #3*

- 2 cups plain nonfat yogurt
- 1 cup thawed frozen orange juice concentrate
- 1 cup raisins
- 4 peeled, cored, chopped apples

Stir all together with a fork until well mixed.

Makes 6 cups

7. *Yogurt-Chive Dressing*

- 1 cup plain nonfat yogurt
- 2 finely chopped scallions
- 6 tablespoons chives
- 2 tablespoons vinegar
- 1/2 teaspoon white pepper
- 1 teaspoon Salt Sub (see page 191) or 1 tablespoon vegetable-broth powder

Mix all ingredients together.

Makes 1 1/2 cups

8. *French Dressing #1*

- 1 cup unsalted tomato juice
- 2 tablespoons rice vinegar
- 1 teaspoon onion flakes
- $^1/_8$ teaspoon sweet basil
- $^1/_8$ teaspoon mustard powder
- $^1/_8$ teaspoon garlic powder
- $^1/_8$ teaspoon pepper

Mix well and chill before serving.

Makes 1 cup

9. *French Dressing #2*

- 1 tablespoon arrowroot
- 2 cups rice vinegar or any other mild vinegar
- 2 cups V-8 juice, preferably unsalted
- 1 cup tomato juice
- $^1/_3$ cup lemon juice
- 3 tablespoons thawed apple juice concentrate
- 3 tablespoons tomato paste
- 1 small chopped onion
- $^1/_2$ chopped green pepper
- 1 teaspoon celery seed
- 1 teaspoon dill seed
- 1 teaspoon paprika
- $^1/_8$ teaspoon cayenne pepper
- 1 teaspoon finely minced parsley

Mix arrowroot with 2 tablespoons cold water to make a paste. Combine remaining ingredients except the parsley in a saucepan. Heat to boiling, then gradually add the arrowroot paste. Cook for 5 more minutes, stirring as needed. Cool and transfer to blender and blenderize. Add parsley and stir. Chill well before serving.

Makes about 6 cups

10. *Tomato Juice Salad Dressing*

- 1 cup unsalted tomato juice
- 1/4 teaspoon lemon juice
- 2 tablespoons finely grated celery
- 1 clove minced garlic
- 1/2 teaspoon oregano
- 1 tablespoon vegetable-broth powder
- 1/2 teaspoon Salt Sub (see page 191)

Shake vigorously in a sealed jar. Refrigerate well before using.

Makes about 1 cup

11. *Spicy Dressing*

- 3/4 cup apple juice
- 1/2 cup cider vinegar
- 2 1/4 teaspoons garlic powder
- 2 1/4 teaspoons cornstarch
- 1 1/2 teaspoons crushed oregano
- 3/4 teaspoon mustard powder
- 3/4 teaspoon paprika
- 1/4 teaspoon ground black pepper

Combine all ingredients in a small saucepan. Bring to a boil. Cook, stirring until thickened, about 2 minutes. Pour into a small bowl. Chill, covered, until ready to use. Mix well before using.

Makes about 1 1/4 cups

12. *Yogurt-Cheese Dressing*

- 1 cup plain nonfat yogurt
- 1/2 cup cider vinegar
- 2 tablespoons grated sapsago cheese
- 1 teaspoon dried parsley
- 1/4 teaspoon garlic powder
- 1/4 teaspoon paprika

Blenderize all ingredients. Chill.

Makes about 1 2/3 cups

13. *Tangy Thousand Island Dressing*

- 1 cup plain nonfat yogurt
- 1/4 cup tomato paste
- 1 teaspoon mustard powder
- 1/2 teaspoon powdered horseradish
- 1/2 teaspoon onion powder
- 1/8 teaspoon pepper
- 1 diced hard-boiled egg white
- 3 tablespoons chopped dill pickles

Combine the ingredients and chill before serving.

Makes about 1 1/2 cups

14. *Nonfat Yogurt-Tomato Dressing*

- 1/2 cup tomato juice
- 1 8-ounce can tomato sauce
- 1 cup plain nonfat yogurt
- 1/2 teaspoon salad herbs
- 1 teaspoon lemon juice or vinegar
- 1 teaspoon diced green chilies
- 1 teaspoon honey
- 1/2 teaspoon dill
- 1/2 teaspoon fresh parsley

Blenderize until smooth. Chill before serving.

Makes about 2 1/2 cups

15. *Italian Dressing*

- 1/4 cup lemon juice
- 1/4 cup vinegar
- 1/4 cup unsweetened apple juice
- 1/2 teaspoon oregano
- 1/2 teaspoon mustard powder
- 1/2 teaspoon garlic powder
- 1/2 teaspoon paprika
- 1/2 teaspoon thyme
- 1/4 teaspoon rosemary

Mix all ingredients in a blender. Chill well before serving.

Makes about 3/4 cup

16. *Creamy Artichoke Dressing*

- 1 cup canned water-packed artichokes
- $^2/_3$ cup nonfat buttermilk
- $1^1/_2$ teaspoons vinegar
- 1 teaspoon diced scallion
- $^1/_4$ teaspoon basil
- $^1/_2$ teaspoon onion powder
- 1 teaspoon crumbled hoop cheese, farmer cheese, or uncreamed cottage cheese

Blenderize all ingredients except the cheese. While the blender is running, add the cheese until the dressing is smooth. Chill well before serving.

Makes about $2^1/_2$ cups

Alfalfa Sprout Dressing

- juice of 3 lemons
- 2 tablespoons honey
- 1 tablespoon granular lecithin
- 1 tablespoon garlic powder or 2 cloves fresh garlic
- 2 tablespoons paprika
- 12 to 16 ounces alfalfa sprouts
- $^2/_3$ cup parsley leaves, finely chopped

Put liquid ingredients in blender first, then spices. While blender is running, gradually add sprouts. If mixture is too thick, add a little water. Then add parsley. Chill.

Tofu Mayonnaise

- 1 pound washed, drained tofu
- $^1/_4$ cup granular lecithin
- $^1/_4$ cup lemon juice or apple cider vinegar
- $^1/_2$ teaspoon Salt Sub (see page 191)
- 1 tablespoon honey
- $^3/_4$ cup food-grade linseed oil

Cut tofu into large chunks and place in blender. Add all remaining ingredients, except $^1/_2$ cup of the oil, and blenderize. With blender at medium-high speed, slowly, drop by drop, add remaining oil. Blend several minutes until very smooth and thick. Chill.

Variation: Add $^1/_2$ teaspoon of garlic powder, dill weed, or tarragon.

Twenty-one Bread Recipes

1. *Basic Oatmeal Muffins*

We've made this recipe number one to emphasize that it should be used often as a source of one of nature's finest grain fibers.

- 2 egg whites
- 2 tablespoons honey
- $^3/_4$ cup plain nonfat yogurt
- $^3/_4$ cup apple or orange juice
- 1 teaspoon baking soda
- $1^3/_4$ cups oatmeal
- $^1/_2$ cup oat bran
- $^1/_2$ cup raisins

Stir all ingredients together, starting from the top of the list and working your way down. Bake in a Pam-sprayed nonstick muffin tin in a preheated 350° oven for 30 minutes or until done.

Variation: For a finer-textured muffin, blenderize oatmeal before adding to recipe.

Makes 1 dozen

2. *Surprise Muffins*

Make Basic Oatmeal Muffin batter, but omit the raisins. Pour half of the normal amount for one muffin into each muffin cup. Then add one or more of the following, and top with the remaining batter. Bake as above.

unsweetened jelly or jam

orange slice and 1 teaspoon of honey

shredded apple and cinnamon

prune and nutmeg

banana slice

dates

figs

blueberries

3. *Fruit-Nut Muffins*

Same high fiber as the Basic Oatmeal Muffins, but less sweet.

- 4 egg whites
- 2 very ripe blenderized bananas
- 3/4 cup nonfat milk, water, or fruit juice
- 1/2 cup ground raw almonds
- 1 teaspoon baking powder
- 1/2 cup carob powder
- 1 3/4–2 cups oatmeal

Beat the egg whites until fluffy. Fold in the bananas, liquid, and almonds. Add the baking powder and carob powder. Slowly add the oatmeal until the mixture is a muffin-batter consistency; it should hold its shape, but still be very moist. This may require 1 3/4 to 2 cups oatmeal, but use more or less as needed. Bake in a Pam-sprayed nonstick muffin tin in a preheated 350° oven for 30 minutes or until done.

Makes 1 dozen

4. *Pita Pocket Bread*

Available in most markets. Stuff with anything you desire (jelly, vegetables, fruit, honey, or beans) or toast and eat plain with your meal.

5. *Seven-Grain Bread*

Available in most health food stores.

6. *Applesauce Cornbread Muffins*

- 2 cups cornmeal mix
- 1 cup whole-wheat flour
- $^{1}/_{4}$ cup thawed frozen apple juice concentrate
- $1^{1}/_{2}$ cups nonfat buttermilk or plain nonfat milk with a little lemon juice added
- 3 stiffly beaten egg whites
- $1^{1}/_{2}$ cups unsweetened applesauce

Mix the dry ingredients. Combine them with the juice and the buttermilk. Fold in the egg whites and the unsweetened applesauce and bake in a preheated 350° oven for 25 minutes.

Variation: Instead of the applesauce, use $1^{1}/_{2}$ cups blueberries, or omit the fruit altogether and add 1 cup corn kernels and $^{1}/_{2}$ cup sautéed onions and green chilies.

7. *Whole-Wheat Bread*

- 1 tablespoon dry yeast
- $^{1}/_{2}$ teaspoon honey
- 2 cups lukewarm water
- $4^{1}/_{2}$ cups whole-wheat flour

Add the yeast and honey to the water. Let ferment about 15 minutes. Combine the water mixture with the flour and knead in large bowl for about 10 minutes. Set the bowl in a warm place and let rise for 45 minutes. Punch down. Place dough in warmed, Pam-sprayed nonstick loaf pan. After loaf has doubled in size, bake for 40 minutes in a preheated 350° oven. Crust should sound hollow when tapped.

8. *Corn Tortillas*

Look for tortillas that are made of corn, water, and lime—and nothing more. Toast in the oven and fill with vegetables. Corn tortillas can also be cut into fourths and toasted in a very hot oven for 5 to 6 minutes to make chips. Season with a no-salt seasoning.

9. *Unsalted RyKrisp*

Available in most markets.

10. *Unsalted Rice Cakes*

Available in most markets. Good with jelly or Nutty Butter (see page 190) or plain with your meal.

11. *Sourdough Bread*

There are very few whole-grain sourdough breads available. It is traditionally made with white flour. Because it contains no fat, sugar, or preservatives, it is acceptable, though a whole-grain bread, because of its higher fiber content, is preferable.

12. *Garlic Bread*

- 1 packet Butter Buds
- 1/2 cup hot water
- 3 large cloves finely minced garlic or 3 tablespoons garlic powder
- 2 tablespoons granular lecithin
- 4 slices bread

Dissolve Butter Buds in the water and add garlic and lecithin. Let marinate in refrigerator awhile. Brush on slices of bread. Broil until toasty. Especially good with sourdough bread.

Makes 4 slices

13. *Cinnamon-Cheese Toast*

- 2 cups hoop cheese or farmer cheese
- 2 tablespoons plain nonfat yogurt
- 4 slices whole-grain bread
- 1 tablespoon cinnamon
- 2 tablespoons date sugar

Cream together the cheese and the yogurt. Spread thickly on the bread slices. Sprinkle with a mixture of the cinnamon and sugar. Broil until bubbly. Serve immediately.

Makes 4 slices

14. *Banana Bread*

- 4 mashed very ripe bananas
- 1 tablespoon honey
- 1 tablespoon baking powder
- 2 teaspoons cinnamon
- 2 cups whole-wheat flour
- 4 egg whites

Optional: $^1/_2$ cup chopped walnuts

Mix the bananas with the honey until creamy. Add the baking powder and cinnamon. Gradually add the flour. Beat the egg whites until fluffy and fold into the flour mixture. If desired, add walnuts. Bake in a nonstick Pam-sprayed loaf pan in a preheated 350° oven for 1 hour or until a toothpick inserted into center comes out clean.

Makes 1 loaf

15. *Oatmeal Bread*

- 1 tablespoon live yeast
- 1/4 cup warm water
- 1 1/2 cups fruit juice
- 1/4 cup honey
- 1/2 teaspoon liquid lecithin
- 1 cup oatmeal
- 3 1/2 cups whole-wheat flour

Dissolve the yeast in the warm water. In a large bowl, mix the fruit juice, honey, and lecithin. Add the oatmeal. Stir in the yeast mixture. Gradually stir in the flour. Knead for 5 minutes on a floured surface. Wash bowl, dry, and spray with Pam. Place the dough in bowl and let rise in a warm place for about an hour. Punch down and put into a lecithin-greased glass loaf pan or nonstick Pam-sprayed loaf pan. Let rise again for one hour. Bake in a preheated 375° oven for 50 minutes.

Makes 1 loaf

16. *Cinnamon Rolls*

- 2 tablespoons yeast
- 1/4 cup warm water
- 1 cup nonfat milk
- 1/2 cup Butter Buds
- 1/4 cup honey
- 4 beaten egg whites
- 2 cups whole-wheat flour
- 2 1/2 cups rice flour

Topping:

- Butter Buds liquid
- honey to taste
- cinnamon to taste

Variation:

- 1/2 cup sesame seeds
- 1/2 cup grated orange rind

Dissolve yeast in the warm water. In a separate bowl, mix the milk, Butter Buds, honey, and egg whites. Gradually add the flours. Knead on floured surface until smooth. Place in a Pam-sprayed bowl to rise for one hour. Punch down and let rise for 10 minutes more. Roll out half of the dough into a rectangle. Spread with filling (see page 272) and roll like a jelly roll.

Cut into 1- to $1^1/_2$-inch slices. Place in a Pam-sprayed nonstick baking pan so that the pieces barely touch. Cover and let rise in a warm place for about 30 minutes or until doubled. (Use the remaining half of the dough in the same way for a second batch.) Bake in a preheated 350° oven for 40 minutes, then for the last 10 minutes, spread liquid Butter Buds on top with honey and cinnamon. Return to oven until browned.

Variation: Sprinkle with sesame seeds and grated orange rind and brown in oven.

Filling:

- 1 cup honey
- 1 tablespoon grated orange rind
- 2 tablespoons orange juice
- 2 teaspoons cinnamon
- $^2/_3$ cup raisins or chopped dates
- $^1/_2$ cup ground sesame seeds or chopped walnuts
- 2 tablespoons dry Butter Buds

Combine all the above ingredients. Use as filling for cinnamon rolls.

Makes 2 dozen (depending on size)

17. *Bread Sticks*

- 2 tablespoons Butter Buds liquid
- 3 tablespoons honey
- 8 slices whole-wheat bread (or other whole-grain bread)
- $^1/_4$ cup sesame seeds

Mix the Butter Buds with the honey. Cut bread into 4 strips per slice. Spread the Butter Buds mixture on the bread and sprinkle with the sesame seeds. Bake in a preheated 400° oven 8 to 10 minutes or until crisp.

Makes 32 sticks

18. *Carrot-Zucchini Bread*

- 4 beaten egg whites
- 3/4 cup honey
- 1 teaspoon liquid lecithin
- 1/2 teaspoon baking soda
- 1/2 teaspoon baking powder
- 1/4 teaspoon ground ginger
- 1 cup grated carrots, loosely packed
- 1 cup grated zucchini, loosely packed
- 1 1/2 cups whole-wheat flour (or mix 3/4 cup whole-wheat flour with another whole-grain flour)

Mix the egg whites with the honey and lecithin. Add the baking soda and powder. Add the ginger. Stir in the carrots and zucchini. Gradually add the flour. Bake in a Pam-sprayed nonstick loaf pan in a preheated 350° oven for 1 hour.

Makes 1 loaf

19. *Irish Soda Bread*

- 2 cups whole-grain flour (rye, graham, whole wheat, buckwheat, or any combination)
- 1 teaspoon baking powder
- 1 tablespoon caraway seeds
- 1/2 teaspoon baking soda
- 1/2 teaspoon cream of tartar
- 6 ounces plain nonfat yogurt (or 2 ounces plain yogurt mixed with 4 ounces nonfat milk)
- 1/2 cup cornmeal

Stir together the flour, baking powder, caraway seeds, baking soda, and cream of tartar. Knead in the yogurt until you can form a ball. Add nonfat milk if needed. Place dough into a cornmeal-sprinkled pie pan. Flatten dough ball and make into a circle approximately 8 inches across. Cut a 1/4-inch-deep **X** into top of dough. Bake in a preheated 400° oven for about 50 minutes.

Makes 1 loaf

20. *Pumpkin or Sweet Potato or Yam Bread*

- 1/3 cup Butter Buds liquid
- 1/2 cup orange or pineapple juice concentrate
- 4 egg whites
- 1 cup mashed cooked pumpkin, sweet potato, or yam
- 1 teaspoon baking soda
- 1 teaspoon cinnamon
- 1/4 teaspoon nutmeg
- 1/8 teaspoon ginger
- 1 3/4 cups whole-wheat flour (or 1 cup whole-wheat mixed with 3/4 cup other whole-grain flour)

Optional: 1/4 cup drained, unsweetened pineapple chunks

Blenderize the Butter Buds with the fruit juice concentrate and egg whites. While the blender is running add the pumpkin, sweet potato, or yam. Add the baking soda, cinnamon, nutmeg, and ginger. Gradually add the flour until of a doughy consistency. If you plan to use the pineapple chunks, add separately; do not blenderize. Bake in a Pam-sprayed nonstick loaf pan in a preheated 350° oven for 45 to 60 minutes or until a toothpick, when inserted into center of loaf, comes out clean.

Makes 1 loaf

21. *Nutty Butter Bread*

Whole grain toast
Nutty Butter (see page 190)

Spread toasted bread with Nutty Butter.

Blueberry Bran Muffins

- 1/2 cup boiling water
- 1 1/2 cups bran
- 1/3 cup honey
- 2 tablespoons granular lecithin
- 2 tablespoons food-grade linseed oil
- 3/4 cup plain nonfat yogurt
- 1 1/4 teaspoons baking soda
- 1 teaspoon Salt Sub (see page 191)
- 1 1/2 cups oat flour or whole-wheat flour
- 3 stiffly beaten egg whites
- 1/2 cup blueberries

Pour boiling water over bran, stir, and set aside for 5 to 10 minutes. Cream together honey, lecithin, and oil. Add yogurt and softened bran. Stir in dry ingredients. Fold in egg whites and blueberries. Pour into a Pam-sprayed nonstick muffin tin 3/4 full. Bake in a preheated 350° oven for 25 minutes.

Makes 1 dozen

Oat-Millet-Rice Muffins

- 1 cup rolled oats
- 1/2 cup millet
- 1/2 cup brown rice
- 1/4 cup honey
- 1/4 cup food-grade linseed oil
- 1/2 teaspoon Salt Sub (see page 191)
- 2 teaspoons baking powder
- 3/4 cup plain nonfat yogurt
- 3 egg whites

Grind oats, millet, and rice in a dry blender, just covering blade, about 1/2 cup grain at a time. Blend honey, oil, Salt Sub, baking powder, and yogurt in blender. Beat egg whites until stiff. Set aside. Stir flours into liquid ingredients and fold in egg whites. Pour into a Pam-sprayed nonstick muffin tin and bake at 375° for 20 to 30 minutes.

Makes 1 dozen

Buckwheat Muffins

- 1½ cups fresh-ground buckwheat flour
- ⅔ cup fresh finely ground walnuts or pecans
- ½ teaspoon Salt Sub (see page 191)
- 2 tablespoons food-grade linseed oil
- 1 tablespoon honey or maple syrup
- 2 tablespoons granular lecithin
- ½ cup soaked raisins
- 1 cup water (more if needed) or thawed frozen apple juice concentrate
- 3 egg whites

Combine all ingredients except egg whites. Whip egg whites last, until stiff. Fold in carefully. Bake in a preheated 425° oven for 20 minutes.

Makes 1 dozen

Caraway-Millet Muffins

- 1 cup hot Nut Milk (see page 292) or hot nonfat milk
- 1 cup millet flour
- 1 tablespoon dry yeast
- ¼ cup warm water
- 1 tablespoon honey
- 1 tablespoon food-grade linseed oil
- 1 egg white
- 1 tablespoon granular lecithin
- 1 teaspoon caraway seeds
- 1 teaspoon Salt Sub (see page 191)
- ¾ cup brown-rice flour

Blend the Nut Milk and the millet flour and let cool. Dissolve the yeast in the water and add to the millet mixture. Let rise 30 minutes or more and add the other ingredients. Blend thoroughly. Pour into muffin tins and bake in a preheated 400° oven for 25 minutes.

Makes 1 dozen

Three Weeks of Dessert Ideas

1. *Carob-Mint Mousse*

- 2 envelopes unflavored gelatin
- 2 tablespoons unsweetened carob powder
- 1 cup thawed frozen apple juice concentrate
- 2 1/2 teaspoons vanilla extract
- 3 1/4 cups nonfat milk
- 1/3 cup dry nonfat milk
- 1/4 teaspoon mint flakes

Optional: fruit slices, fresh mint

Place the gelatin and carob powder in a large bowl, add 1/4 cup of the apple juice, and mix well. Heat the remaining apple juice and vanilla extract to a boil in a saucepan and turn down the heat. Add the gelatin and carob mixture and stir constantly over low heat for about 5 minutes. Refrigerate until cool. Place milk (both dry and liquid), mint flakes, and gelatin mixture in a blender, half at a time if necessary, and blend. When fluffy and light, transfer to a mixing bowl and chill until cold and thickened—not frozen. Whip with an electric mixer. Return to the freezer. Whip once more before serving. Do not freeze. Garnish with fruit slices, if desired, or a sprig of fresh mint.

Makes about 5 1/2-cup servings

2. *Baked Apple*

- 1 cored tart apple
- 1 tablespoon raisins
- 1 teaspoon thawed orange juice concentrate
- 1/8 teaspoon cinnamon

Fill the apple with the remaining mixed ingredients. Place in an ovenproof dish with 1 inch of water in it. Cover. Bake in a preheated 400° oven for 40 to 60 minutes or until apple is soft.

Serves 1

3. *Pumpkin Ice Cream*

- 1 package unflavored gelatin
- 1/4 cup hot water
- 1 cup frozen orange juice concentrate
- 1 1-pound can unsweetened pumpkin
- 1/2 teaspoon ginger
- 1/2 teaspoon cinnamon
- 1/2 teaspoon nutmeg
- 1/2 cup nonfat milk

Dissolve gelatin in water. Blenderize orange juice with pumpkin and seasonings. Add milk. Put in a shallow pan and freeze. Stir often.

Serves 6 to 8

4. *Fresh Fruit Ice Cream*

- 3 very ripe bananas
- 1 pint strawberries
- 6 ounces nonfat yogurt

Combine the ingredients in a blender until smooth. Freeze in a loaf pan until firm. Scrape into an ice cream scoop to serve.

Serves 6 to 8

5. *Cheesy-Lemon Pie*

- 1 pound uncreamed cottage cheese
- 1 cup nonfat milk
- 6 ounces thawed frozen pineapple juice concentrate
- 1 teaspoon vanilla extract
- 1 teaspoon lemon extract
- 4 stiffly beaten egg whites
- 1/2 cup Grape-Nuts cereal
- pineapple juice or water

Blenderize first 5 ingredients. Fold the mixture into the egg whites. Pour into a Pam-sprayed pie pan that is lined with 1/4-inch-thick

Grape-Nuts moistened with pineapple juice or water. Bake in a preheated 350° oven for 1 hour. Serve warm or chilled.

Makes 1 pie

6. *Apple Crisp*

- 4 cups pared sliced apples
- 1 tablespoon lemon juice
- 1 teaspoon cinnamon
- 1½ cups natural flake cereal
- ½ cup whole-wheat flour
- ¼ cup date sugar
- ⅓ cup chopped almonds
- 2 tablespoons Butter Buds liquid

Fill a Pam-sprayed pie plate with the apples. Sprinkle with the lemon juice and cinnamon. Crush the cereal with a rolling pin and mix with the flour, sugar, almonds, and Butter Buds liquid. Sprinkle the cereal mixture over the apples. Bake in a preheated 350° oven for 30 minutes.

Makes 1 pie

7. *Frozen Banana Pie*

- ¾ cup oatmeal
- ¼ cup raw unhulled sesame seeds
- ½ cup pureed dates
- 5 very ripe bananas

Optional: 1 tablespoon carob powder, 1 teaspoon honey

Blenderize the oatmeal with the seeds and knead in the dates. (The mixture should hold together but still be somewhat dry.) Press into a pie plate. In a clean blender, blenderize 4 bananas. (At this time half of this mixture can be set aside and used to make a "chocolate" mixture by adding the carob powder and honey. This is used as a decorative border on the pie.) Pour the plain banana mixture into the pie crust. Slice the fifth banana in a circle pattern on top. If you added carob and honey to half the banana mixture, pour the chocolate border. Freeze overnight. Thaw very slightly before serving, being careful not to overthaw, or pie will become runny.

Makes 1 pie

8. *Berry Pie*

- 3 tablespoons tapioca granules
- 1½ cups berry juice, unsweetened (boysenberry, blackberry, or grape)
- 1 teaspoon vanilla
- 2 apples or pears, peeled and sliced
- 1 cup berries
- ¼ cup raisins
- ¾ cup oatmeal
- ¼ cup raw unhulled sesame seeds
- 1 teaspoon cinnamon

In a Pam-sprayed glass pie pan, mix the tapioca with the berry juice and vanilla. Layer the apple or pear slices to cover the pan. Next layer the berries. Sprinkle with the raisins. On top, sprinkle a blenderized mixture of the oatmeal, seeds, and cinnamon. Bake in a preheated 350° oven for 30 minutes. Serve warm.

Makes 1 pie

9. *Peach Pie*

- 2 tablespoons grain beverage coffee substitute, dry
- ¾ cup Grape-Nuts
- 4 tablespoons fruit juice
- 2 tablespoons vanilla extract
- 2 cups apple or pear juice
- 2 tablespoons tapioca granules
- 1 package frozen peaches or 3 fresh large peaches

Make a crust by pouring a mixture of the first three ingredients into a Pam-sprayed pie pan. Mix the next three ingredients and pour into the pie crust. Layer the peach slices on top. Top all with more cereal and cinnamon, if desired. Bake in a preheated 350° oven for 45 minutes. Cool before serving.

Makes 1 pie

10. *Pumpkin Pie*

- 1 16-ounce can unsweetened pumpkin
- 1 6-ounce can thawed frozen apple- or pineapple-juice concentrate
- 1 teaspoon cinnamon
- 1/4 teaspoon allspice
- 1/4 teaspoon ginger
- 1/4 teaspoon cloves or nutmeg
- 1 teaspoon vanilla extract
- 1/2 cup crushed Grape-Nuts cereal
- 1–2 tablespoons fruit juice or water
- 6 stiffly beaten egg whites

Blenderize all but the cereal, fruit juice or water, and egg whites. Line a Pam-sprayed pie pan with the Grape-Nuts, then moisten with the fruit juice or water. In a mixing bowl, fold the egg whites into the blenderized mixture. Pour into the pie pan. Bake in a preheated 350° oven for 1 hour or until a toothpick inserted into the center shows it is firm but still moist.

Makes 1 pie

11. *"Ice Cream"*

Very ripe bananas

Peel ripe bananas and freeze overnight in a plastic bag. Run the frozen banana through a juicer that has a spout that shoots out the pulp. The bananas will be the consistency of soft-serve ice cream.

Variations: For flavors, freeze other ripe fruits such as strawberries, peaches, apricots, or blueberries and run through the juicer along with the banana.

12. *Chewy Oat-Orange Drops*

- 1 cup oatmeal
- 2 cups orange juice
- 1 tablespoon tapioca granules
- 1 cup whole-wheat flour
- 2 tablespoons honey
- 2 tablespoons whey powder
- 2 tablespoons grated orange rind
- 1/2 teaspoon cinnamon
- 3 teaspoons baking powder
- 1 teaspoon liquid lecithin

Mix the oatmeal with the orange juice and tapioca and let stand. After 15 minutes add the other ingredients. Beat with a fork until well mixed. Drop by the tablespoon onto a Pam-sprayed nonstick cookie sheet. Bake in a preheated 300° oven for about 20 minutes or until done.

Makes about 2 dozen

13. *Fruit Tapioca*

- 1/4 cup tapioca granules
- 2 cups orange juice
- 1/2 cup orange juice concentrate

Blend tapioca with orange juices. Let stand for 5 minutes. Bring to boil over medium heat, stirring often. Cool for 20 minutes. Stir well. Serve warm or cold.

Makes 6 1/2-cup servings

14. *Cherry Pie*

- 2½ tablespoons tapioca granules
- ⅛ teaspoon mace
- ½ cup concentrated orange juice
- 3 cups sweet cherries
- ¼ teaspoon almond extract
- 1¼ cups crushed Grape-Nuts cereal
- 1–2 tablespoons fruit juice or water

Blend together the tapioca, mace, orange juice, and let stand. Stir in the cherries after 15 minutes, and the almond extract. Pour into a Pam-sprayed pie pan lined with ¾ cup Grape-Nuts. Top with remaining cereal that has soaked 1 hour in fruit juice or water. Bake in a preheated 425° oven for about 50 minutes.

Note: Cherries are available in most markets year round in the frozen foods section. Look for the unsweetened sweet cherries.

Makes 1 pie

15. *Fresh Fruit Salad*

- banana
- papaya
- strawberries
- seedless grapes
- pineapple

Optional: slivered almonds

Wash and cut up fresh fruits. Toss with the natural juice of the fruits or add additional unsweetened fruit juice. Garnish with a sprig of fresh mint. If desired, toss in almonds.

16. *Sesame Balls*

- 1 cup oatmeal, ground coarsely in a grinder or blender
- ½ cup unhulled raw sesame seeds
- date paste (pureed dates)

Form the oats and seeds into balls by kneading with the date paste.

Makes about 2 dozen balls

17. *Stewed Prunes and Apricots*

- 1 16-ounce bag dried prunes
- 1 16-ounce bag dried apricots

Optional: cinnamon, cloves

Place the fruit in a large pot and cover with water. Simmer on very low heat for 1 hour. Remove from heat and spin lid of the pot to seal. Let sit overnight. Put into jars and store in the refrigerator. Serve warm, before putting into the refrigerator; serve remaining fruit cold. If desired, dish may be seasoned with cinnamon and cloves.

Makes about 4 cups

18. *Banana Boats*

- 1 ripe banana
- 2 tablespoons plain nonfat yogurt
- 1 tablespoon berries
- 1 tablespoon honey
- 1–2 teaspoons slivered almonds

Slice one banana per person, in half, lengthwise. Place in a long dish. Place two portions of yogurt in between halves. Top with berries. Drizzle with honey. Sprinkle with almond slivers. Serve cold.

Serves 1

19. *Banana Pudding*

(Or use as a pie filling.)

- 1 quart nonfat milk
- 1/2 cup honey
- 6 tablespoons arrowroot
- 1 teaspoon vanilla
- 1 1/2 cups mashed ripe banana
- 1/2 cup boiling water
- 2 tablespoons agar

Blenderize the milk, honey, arrowroot, and vanilla. Heat until thick. Add the milk mixture to the mashed banana. In another pan, heat the water and agar. Add to the banana-milk mixture. Chill and serve.

Makes 15 1/2-cup servings

20. *Carob Brownies*

- 4 egg whites
- 2/3 cup honey
- 1/2 cup Butter Buds liquid
- 1 teaspoon vanilla
- 1 mashed banana
- 1 teaspoon baking soda
- 1/3 cup sifted carob powder
- 3/4 cup water
- 1 cup whole-wheat flour
- 1/2 cup broken walnut pieces

Beat the egg whites lightly. Add the honey, Butter Buds, vanilla, and banana. Mix well. Add the baking soda and carob powder. Stir in the water, and alternately add the flour and walnut pieces. Bake in a lecithin-greased lightly floured 13-inch-by-9-inch nonstick baking dish at 350° for 20 to 25 minutes. Watch for burning!

Note: For carob cake, double the recipe and bake in cake pans for 40 minutes.

Makes 1 dozen

21. *Rice Pudding*

- $1\frac{1}{2}$ cups nonfat milk
- 4 egg whites
- 2 tablespoons honey
- $\frac{1}{2}$ teaspoon nutmeg
- 1 teaspoon cinnamon
- 1 tablespoon tapioca granules
- 2 cups cooked brown rice
- 1 cup raisins

In a double boiler, heat the milk. In a bowl, beat egg whites lightly. Add the honey, nutmeg, cinnamon, and tapioca to the egg whites. Slowly add the egg white mixture to the hot milk, stirring constantly about 10 minutes or until mixture starts to thicken. Remove from heat and add the rice. Mix well. Add the raisins. Mix well. Pour into a Pam-sprayed nonstick 2-quart baking dish. Bake in a preheated 350° oven for 15 minutes or until set. Serve warm or cold.

Makes about 5 cups

Candy Supreme

- 1 cup honey
- $\frac{1}{4}$ cup carob powder
- $\frac{1}{2}$ cup ground walnuts
- $\frac{1}{2}$ cup ground sunflower seeds
- $\frac{1}{2}$ cup chopped dates
- $\frac{1}{2}$ cup chopped dried apricot or apple

Optional: $\frac{1}{2}$ cup sesame seeds

Cream together honey and carob powder. Add nuts and sunflower seeds. Stir in dried fruits. Shape into $\frac{1}{2}$- to $\frac{3}{4}$-inch balls and roll in sesame seeds or spread in a Pam-sprayed nonstick cake pan and sprinkle sesame seeds over all. Chill and serve.

Makes 2 dozen balls

Pineapple-Mint Tingle

- 6 cups fresh pineapple chunks
- 6 tablespoons shredded fresh mint leaves
- honey to taste

Put in covered glass dish and chill for several hours. Serve in fancy dessert cups and garnish with a sprig of fresh mint.

Serves 6

Apricot Cloud

- 1 cup dried apricots
- 1/4 cup honey
- 6 egg whites

Cover apricots with water and soak overnight. Blenderize apricots with honey. Beat egg whites until stiff and fold in apricot mixture. Gently mound mixture into a Pam-sprayed nonstick baking dish and bake in a preheated 375° oven for 30 minutes or until firm.

Serves 6

Yogurt Ice Cream

- 1 cup plain nonfat yogurt
- 2 cups fresh fruit (strawberry, peach, blueberry, or mango)
- 1/3 cup honey
- 1 tablespoon lemon juice

Blend all together and freeze in a shallow pan or, for best results, an ice cream freezer. Can take out after several hours, reblend, and return to freezer till firm.

Serves 2 to 4

Cantaloupe Circles

- 1 cantaloupe
- strawberries, raspberries, or cherries
- plain nonfat yogurt
- sunflower seeds

Peel a whole cantaloupe. Cut in half and remove seeds. Slice into circles. Fill center with berries and top with a dollop of yogurt and a sprinkle of sunflower seeds.

Ambrosia Delight

- 2 cups sliced ripe bananas
- 2 cups fresh pineapple chunks
- 1 peeled, seeded, and cubed papaya

Dressing:

- $^1/_2$ cup plain nonfat yogurt
- juice of 1 orange
- 2 tablespoons honey

Make a dressing by combining yogurt, orange juice, and honey. Pour over mixed fruits.

Pineapple Upside-down Cake

- 2 tablespoons food-grade linseed oil
- 2 tablespoons liquid lecithin
- $^1/_4$ cup honey
- $^1/_4$ cup date sugar
- 4–6 fresh or canned pineapple rings, $^1/_4$-inch thick
- 2 teaspoons vanilla
- 1 cup honey
- $^1/_4$ cup food-grade linseed oil
- $^1/_2$ cup water
- $^1/_2$ cup plain nonfat yogurt
- 3 cups whole-wheat pastry flour
- 4 teaspoons low-sodium baking powder
- $^1/_2$ teaspoon Salt Sub (see page 191)

Spray a 9-inch nonstick baking pan with Pam. Melt first 3 ingredients in small saucepan. Pour into baking dish and sprinkle evenly with the date sugar. Arrange pineapple rings in the syrup.

Blend the next 5 ingredients well, using either a blender or an electric mixer. Next add dry ingredients and blend until smooth. Pour over pineapple rings and spread evenly. Bake for 45 minutes in a preheated 350° oven. Turn upside down onto a tray or platter as soon as it comes out of the oven.

Serves 4–6

Three Weeks of Beverage Ideas

1. *Herb Tea*

Prepare as per package instructions and sweeten with honey.
Serve hot or iced.
Especially good tasting for beginners:
- lemon grass
- mint
- orange spice

Especially good for the heart:
- hawthorne berry

Especially good for blood sugar:
- licorice root

2. *Perrier Water, Seltzer, or Club Soda*

To Perrier water, seltzer, or club soda, add ice cubes made of frozen fruit juice. Pineapple juice, orange juice, or lemon juice are excellent choices.
Good for entertaining.

3. *Fruit Juice*

Any of a number of bottled, frozen, or fresh unsweetened fruit juices, such as:

- apple
- orange
- prune
- papaya
- pineapple
- papaya-pineapple
- boysenberry-apple
- pear
- blackberry
- grape
- pear-apple

4. *Grain Beverage Coffee Substitute (Pero, Duram, Roastaroma, Pioneer)*

An instant hot grain beverage you drink instead of coffee.

5. *Vegetable Juice*

Make your own or buy fresh in your health food store; canned varieties contain too much salt. Use carrot juice as a base if you prefer your vegetable juice to taste sweeter. Add parsley, celery, cucumber, green pepper, or beet juice.

6. *Banana Smoothie*

1 cup orange juice
1 ripe, peeled banana
3 pitted dates

Optional: ice cubes

Blenderize fruits together, starting with the orange juice. Serve cold. For a thicker, richer, colder drink, freeze the ripe, peeled banana first. Or use $^{3}/_{4}$ cup orange juice and add several ice cubes while blending.

Makes 1 glass

7. *Hot Caroboca*

- 1 tablespoon carob powder
- 1 teaspoon honey
- 1/4 teaspoon vanilla
- 1/8 teaspoon cinnamon
- 1 cup heated nonfat milk

Blenderize carob powder, honey, vanilla, and cinnamon. Add the carob mixture to the heated milk. Serve hot.

Makes 1 glass

8. *Fruit Punch*

- 1 pint berry juice or grape juice
- 4 cups orange juice
- 1/2 cup lemon juice
- 1 pint club soda or Perrier
- fresh orange, lemon, and lime slices

Optional: frozen fruit juice ice cubes (pineapple, orange, lemon, or apple)

Mix the juices and club soda or Perrier together. Decorate with the citrus fruit slices. Serve cold.

Optional: Instead of the citrus fruit slices, float frozen fruit juice ice cubes in the punch bowl.

Makes about 3 pints

9. *Hot Apple Cider*

- 1 gallon unsweetened apple cider or apple juice
- 1 teaspoon whole cloves
- 4 cinnamon sticks
- 1 teaspoon whole allspice

Heat the apple juice for 10 minutes. Add the spices. Heat an additional 10 minutes. Strain out the spices. Serve hot.

Makes 1 gallon

10. *Monkey Milk*

1 cup nonfat milk
2 tablespoons plain nonfat yogurt
$^1/_2$ teaspoon vanilla
1 large ripe banana

Blenderize all together. Serve ice-cold.

Makes 1 glass

11. *Natural Soda*

4 tablespoons orange juice concentrate
1 cup Perrier or club soda

Stir or shake together. Serve with frozen fruit juice ice cubes.

Makes 1 glass

12. *Nut Milk*

1 cup blanched raw almonds
1 pint water

Blenderize the almonds with the water. Add more water if necessary to achieve the consistency of a rich, thick milk. Refrigerate and use on cereal or like milk.

Variation: Use sunflower or sesame seeds instead of almonds.

Makes $1^1/_2$ pints

13. *Nonfat Milk*

Limit to 8 ounces a day.

14. *Yogurt Drink*

- 8 ounces plain nonfat yogurt
- 1/4 cup pineapple juice (or pineapple chunks in their own juice, or 2 tablespoons thawed pineapple juice concentrate)

Stir together. Serve cold.

Makes 1 cup

15. *Tea and Juice Blend*

This is an excellent way to use leftover herb tea.

- 1 cup herb tea
- 1–2 cups fruit juices

Mix together. Almost anything goes, but you may not like prune or cranberry juice in this drink.

Makes 1 to 3 cups

16. *Strawberry Shake*

- 1 cup orange juice
- 1/2 cup frozen whole unsweetened strawberries
- 1/8 teaspoon almond extract

Blenderize and serve cold.

Makes 1 glass

17. *Banana-Nut Milk*

1 ripe banana
1 cup Nut Milk (see page 292)
1/8 teaspoon vanilla
1/8 teaspoon cinnamon

Blenderize all together. Serve ice-cold.

Makes 1 glass

18. *Tomato Juice Cocktail*

1 pint water
1 can unsalted tomato paste
1 pint mixed fresh vegetable juices (carrot, celery, parsley, beet)
4 tablespoons vinegar
2 tablespoons lemon juice
2 tablespoons vegetable-broth powder
parsley or mint

Blenderize all ingredients except garnish and chill. Shake well before serving. Garnish with a sprig of parsley or mint.

Makes 2 pints

19. *Thick Apple Drink*

1 cup apple juice
1 ripe peeled cored pear, preferably Bartlett
1 ice cube

Blenderize until smooth. Serve ice-cold.

Makes 1 glass

20. *Fruity Float*

- unsweetened white grape juice
- frozen seedless green grapes
- frozen strawberries
- frozen pineapple chunks

In a punch bowl or individual glasses, float the frozen fruits—use instead of ice cubes—when serving.

21. *Lemon Cooler*

- 2 cups apple juice
- 1/4 cup fresh lemon juice
- 1 tablespoon thawed frozen pineapple juice concentrate

Blenderize ingredients and serve ice-cold.

Makes 2 glasses

22. *Lemon Froth*

- 1/2 cup plain nonfat yogurt
- juice of 1/2 lemon
- 1 tablespoon pure maple syrup or honey
- 1/2–1 cup crushed ice or 1/2 cup cold water and 4 ice cubes

Blenderize ingredients and serve immediately.

Makes 1 to 2 glasses

Three Weeks of Brown Bag Meals

1. *Bakon, Lettuce, and Tomato Sandwich*

Per sandwich:

- 2 slices toasted whole-grain bread
- 1 tablespoon Miracle Blend Dressing (see page 188)
- 1 large leaf lettuce
- 2 large tomato slices
- Bakon seasoning (see page 186)

Toast the bread. Spread with the dressing. Sprinkle liberally with Bakon seasoning. Arrange with the tomato and lettuce.

2. *Egg-White Salad Sandwich*

Filling:

- 12 chopped hard-boiled egg whites
- 2 stalks chopped celery
- 1/4 cup chopped scallions
- 1/4 cup chopped green pepper
- 1/4 teaspoon cayenne pepper
- 1 tablespoon chopped parsley
- 1/4 teaspoon mustard powder
- 1 teaspoon vegetable-broth powder
- 1/2 cup Miracle Blend Dressing (see page 188)

Combine all ingredients except the dressing. Add dressing a little at a time until the desired moistness is reached. You may need more or less dressing than the recipe indicates.

Serves 6

3. *Pita Sandwich*

Per sandwich:

1 pita pocket bread
1 teaspoon natural prepared mustard or Tofu Mayonnaise (see page 265)
alfalfa sprouts
thin cucumber slices
tomato slices
chives
lettuce
raw hulled sunflower seeds

Open the pocket bread and spread inside with the mustard or Tofu Mayonnaise. Fill with the vegetables and seeds.

4. *Nutty Butter and Jelly Sandwich*

Per sandwich:

2 slices whole-grain bread, toasted or plain
2 tablespoons Nutty Butter (see page 190)
2 tablespoons jelly (see page 188)

Spread the bread with the Nutty Butter and jelly. Or mash fresh ripe fruit with 1 teaspoon honey and use as jelly.

5. *Grilled Banana and Honey Sandwich*

Per sandwich:

1 ripe banana
1 tablespoon honey
2 slices whole-grain bread

Optional: cinnamon

Mash the banana with fork. Spread thickly on bread. Drizzle with honey. Sprinkle with cinnamon, if desired. Grill under broiler until bubbly. Pack in foil.

6. *Bean Burgers*

- 3/4 cup cooked garbanzos
- 1/3 cup cooked kidney beans
- 1/2 cup cooked brown rice
- 1 chopped onion
- 1 grated carrot
- 1 stalk chopped celery
- 1 tablespoon Salt Sub (see page 191)
- 3 tablespoons brewer's yeast
- 4 beaten egg whites

Optional: tomato sauce

Combine the beans, rice, onion, carrot, and celery in food processor or blender for an instant (leave chunky, but well blended). Add the Salt Sub, yeast, and egg whites with a fork to blend well. Form into patties and brown on a Pam-sprayed nonstick griddle in some tomato sauce if desired. Serve hot or cold.

Serves 4

7. *Lentil-Spread Sandwich*

- 1 cup cooked lentils
- 1 cooked carrot
- 1 small tomato
- 1 tablespoon cider
- 2 tablespoons vegetable-broth powder
- 1 teaspoon Salt Sub (see page 191)
- 1 tablespoon natural prepared mustard
- tomato juice
- lettuce leaves
- tomato slices

Blenderize all but the lettuce and tomato until smooth. Add tomato juice as needed to keep from being too dry. Use liberally as sandwich filling along with the lettuce and tomatoes.

Serves 4

8. *Falafel Burgers*

- 1 package falafel mix (purchase at a health food store)
- water
- 1 tablespoon unrefined sesame oil
- lettuce leaves
- tomato slices

Mix the dry falafel mix with an equal amount of water in a large bowl and add the sesame oil. Let set 15 to 30 minutes. (*Note:* If you accidentally add too much water and the mix is watery and will not form a patty, add whole-wheat flour until the proper consistency is reached.) With an ice cream scoop, drop onto a Pam-sprayed cookie sheet using about 1/2 cup of the mixture per patty. Flatten. Bake in a preheated 400° oven about 30 minutes or until browned. Serve on any kind of bread with Tahini Sauce (see below), tomato slices, and lettuce leaves.

Serves 7 to 10

Tahini Sauce

- 1/4 cup tahini, drained of oil
- 3/4 cup tomato juice
- 1 clove fresh minced garlic
- 1–2 tablespoons lemon juice

Combine tahini with tomato juice. Season with garlic and lemon juice. You will end up with a catsup appearance and consistency though a different flavor.

9. *Yogurt Meal*

- 8 ounces nonfat yogurt
- 1 tablespoon natural honey
- 1/2 cup mashed fruit (berries, peaches, apricots, pineapple, or your favorite fruit)

Using a fork, mix the yogurt with the honey and fruit. Keep refrigerated until serving.

Serves 1

10. *Rice and Vegetables in a Thermos*

- 1/4 cup brown rice
- 1 cup water
- 1 10-ounce package mixed vegetables
- 2 tablespoons vegetable-broth powder

Cook the rice in the water for 30 minutes. Add the vegetables and cook 15 minutes more, adding the vegetable-broth powder the last 5 minutes of cooking. Pour into a preheated 16-ounce thermos.

Note: To preheat a thermos, fill it with boiling water and let it set a minute. Empty the water and fill immediately with the food.

Serves 1

11. *Take-Along Beans in a Thermos*

- 1/2 cup beans (kidney, pinto, lentils, or garbanzos)
- 1 1/2 cups water
- 1 large sliced carrot
- 1/4 teaspoon thyme
- 1 teaspoon Salt Sub (see page 191)

Cook the beans in the water for 30 minutes (20 minutes for lentils, 45 minutes for garbanzos), add the carrot and seasonings, and cook 20 minutes more. Pour into a preheated 16-ounce thermos (see page

300). Beans should still be slightly *al dente,* as the thermos will complete the softening process.

Serves 1

12. *Mushroom Supreme*

- 1 pound fresh mushrooms, washed, dried, and peeled if needed
- 1 bunch minced scallions or medium Bermuda onion
- 1 diced red bell pepper
- 4 diced medium tomatoes
- 2 diced celery stalks
- 1 tablespoon vegetable-broth powder
- 1 clove crushed garlic
- 1/3 cup fresh minced parsley
- juice of 1 large lemon (or 2 small)
- 2 tablespoons food-grade linseed oil

Optional: 1 teaspoon fresh basil and 1/2 cup diced jicama

Mix ingredients together. If desired, stir in basil and jicama. Chill.

Serves 2 to 4

13. *Microwave Meal*

If a microwave oven is available to the brown-bagger, frozen vegetables, such as corn on the cob, mixed vegetables, broccoli, or cauliflower, sealed in their original plastic bags, can be cooked in a microwave oven in the time suggested on the package. Leftover casseroles, rice, or pasta may also be reheated in the same manner.

14. *Nutritional Bars*

- 2 egg whites
- 1/2 cup Butter Buds liquid
- 2/3 cup thawed frozen fruit juice concentrate
- 1/2 teaspoon baking soda
- 1 teaspoon cinnamon
- 1/2 teaspoon coriander
- 1/8 teaspoon cloves
- 1/2 cup bran
- 1 cup whole-wheat flour
- 1 1/2 cups rolled oats
- 1/2 cup raisins
- 1/4 cup chopped raw unsalted nuts
- 1 1/2 cups chopped apples (or mixture of fruits, such as peaches, bananas, apricots, and prunes)

Cream together the egg whites, Butter Buds, and fruit juice. Add the baking soda, cinnamon, coriander, and cloves. Beat well. Gradually add the bran, flour, and oats. Mix well. Add the raisins, nuts, and fruits. Press dough onto a Pam-sprayed nonstick cookie sheet. Bake in a preheated 350° oven for 20 minutes or until done. Cut into bars. Pack several nutritional bars with a thermos of nonfat milk and some fresh fruit.

Makes 1 dozen large bars

15. *Celery with Nutty Butter*

- 6–8 celery stalks
- 1 serving of Nutty Butter (see page 190)

Fill the celery stalks with the Nutty Butter. Keep refrigerated until serving.

Serves 4

16. *Veggie Salad Spread*

- 2 grated raw carrots
- 3 grated raw zucchini
- 1/2 cup finely chopped parsley
- 1/2 cup finely chopped pecans
- 1/2 cup finely chopped sunflower seeds

Moisten vegetables with Creamy French Dressing (see below). Then add blenderized pecans and seeds. Serve on whole-grain bread or crackers, in pita bread, or on a bed of crisp greens.

Serves 4 to 6

Creamy French Dressing

- 1 packet Hain's French dressing mix
- 1/4 cup apple cider vinegar or fresh lemon juice
- 2/3 cup food-grade linseed oil
- 1/2 cup plain nonfat yogurt
- 1 tablespoon granular lecithin

Blenderize and chill.
Variation: Reduce oil to 1/3 cup and increase yogurt to 1 cup.

Serves 4 to 8

17. *Mustard Vegetable Sandwich*

- 2 slices whole-grain bread
- 1 teaspoon natural prepared mustard or Tofu Mayonnaise (see page 265)
- 1 tablespoon chopped mushrooms
- 2–3 tomato slices
- 1 large lettuce leaf
- 1 tablespoon chopped scallions
- 3 cucumber slices
- 1 tablespoon alfalfa sprouts
- 1 pinch Salt Sub (see page 191)

Spread whole-grain bread with mustard or Tofu Mayonnaise. Layer with the vegetables. Sprinkle with the Salt Sub.

18. *Tabouli*

This is a very satisfying meal in itself. Bulgur wheat that has been parboiled and cracked still retains all of the nutritional benefits of the whole grain.

- $1\frac{1}{4}$ cups uncooked bulgur
- 3 chopped scallions
- 1 cup minced fresh parsley
- 3 peeled finely chopped tomatoes
- juice of two lemons
- $\frac{1}{4}$ cup food-grade linseed oil
- Salt Sub (see page 191) to taste
- tomato wedges
- 1 slice Bermuda onion

Pour 3 cups boiling water over bulgur. Let it stand for 1 hour or until grain is light and fluffy. Press out excess water through a colander. Season with the remaining ingredients. Chill several hours before serving. Serve on a bed of crisp chilled greens and garnish with tomato wedges and an onion slice.

19. *Grilled Cheese and Pear Sandwich*

- 2 slices whole-grain bread
- $\frac{1}{2}$ peeled sliced pear
- 1 teaspoon grated sapsago cheese

Place a thin layer of the pears on the bread slices. Grate the cheese over the top. Grill until bubbly. To pack, wrap in foil.

Serves 1

20. *Barley Soup*

- 1 chopped carrot
- 1 chopped onion
- 1 stalk chopped celery
- 2 tablespoons whole-wheat flour
- 3 cups vegetable stock
- 8 peeled tomatoes
- 1 clove minced garlic
- 1 teaspoon basil
- 1 teaspoon oregano
- 1/8 teaspoon white pepper
- 1 tablespoon thawed frozen apple juice concentrate
- 1 1/2 cups cooked barley
- 3 cups nonfat milk or vegetable stock

Sauté the carrot, onion, and celery in water. Add flour and mix. Add the stock, tomatoes, garlic, basil, oregano, pepper, and apple juice concentrate. Simmer for half an hour. Blenderize and return to pan. Add the barley and milk or remaining stock. Reheat, but don't boil. Pour into preheated thermos (see page 300).

Serves 6 to 8

21. *Skim-Milk Ricotta Sandwich*

- 2 tablespoons skim-milk ricotta cheese, crumbled
- 2 slices whole-grain bread
- chopped dates

Spread a thick layer of the ricotta on the bread. Sprinkle with the dates. (Or toast the bread first.) Pack in foil. Can be broiled or warmed before eating. The sandwich can also be broiled or heated in a microwave.

Serves 1

Companion Foods

Along with the main dish, pack one or more of the following:

- bread or toast
- fresh fruit
- raisins, dates, figs, or other dried fruit
- fruit juice or nonfat milk
- vegetable sticks (carrot, celery, cucumber, or your favorite)
- alfalfa sprouts packed separately for freshness

PART IV
Patient Testimonials

Case History

Gene Raymond *Jackson, California*

In September of 1979, I began experiencing some pain in the throat area and across to the upper arms. This began appearing most often about 11:00 P.M., four hours after dinner.

I consulted my regular doctor, a general practitioner, whom I had been seeing at least three times a year for a period of six years. I had experienced high blood pressure for about three years and was under stress test. The results were rather inconclusive. He recommended that I quit smoking and divest myself of some of my corporate duties. He prescribed additional medication for the high blood pressure. I followed his recommendations, and although the pains subsided, they did not disappear completely.

Toward the middle of October 1979, the pains returned in increased intensity and I began using Nitro Salve regularly and some additional medication. I also was examined by a team of cardiac specialists, and it was recommended that if the pains continued, I should have an angiogram.

The first part of November 1979 was quite unbearable as the pains became so severe that I could not move my arms to take the nitro pills. As a result, after additional tests, I was scheduled for the angiogram. It was performed on a Thursday morning, and the results were given to me the following day. The report was that I had three blockages varying from 55 percent to 80 percent and that a triple bypass should be performed Monday morning. It was at this point that I was introduced to the surgeon who would perform the operation. He then explained the routine to me.

This was quite a blow because at the age of sixty-four, the night after the angiogram was the first night I had ever spent in a hospital. I continued to ask for more information regarding an alternate, such as treatment, medication, etc., but was informed that the operation was vital.

I became very apprehensive. I had a feeling I was making an appointment for a haircut rather than having my heart subjected to what appeared to me was a very severe experience. I was in a position that I frankly feel a person with the limited medical knowledge, as I had at the time, is unable to evaluate or cope with intelligently.

Two fortunate things occurred Saturday while in the hospital. I received a visit from my podiatrist and friend, Dr. Hallmeyer of Millbrae, California. I spoke to her of my apprehension. Dr. Hallmeyer suggested that I investigate the program offered by Dr. Whitaker at the National Heart and Diabetes Treatment Institute. She had attended a seminar given by him and was very impressed. The second thing was that I developed a severe cold, and it was determined that I should postpone the operation for a few days until my cold had improved.

I returned home, and after two days of recovering from the cold, I contacted Dr. Whitaker and explained fully what had transpired during the past few months. After answering several questions and conversations between Dr. Whitaker and my doctors, Dr. Whitaker suggested that if I felt capable of doing so, I should come down to the Institute for further examinations and discussions.

Mrs. Raymond and I drove down to the Institute in easy stages as I experienced several angina attacks during the trip. We arrived Sunday afternoon and we were greeted by Dr. Whitaker. After a short period of settling ourselves in our room, I returned to his office for an examination. My medical records had been forwarded to the Institute and upon completion of a thorough examination, Dr. Whitaker spoke to Mrs. Raymond and me and informed us of his conclusions.

We had a decision to make as he did not rule out the possibility of the bypass and that in my case, delay could entail a certain amount of risk, but if we decided to go ahead with his program, he would personally do everything he possibly could to minimize the risk and supervise the treatment. He suggested we consider the problem and let him know Monday at breakfast.

We discussed it at length that evening, and as we were quite impressed with the sincerity and thoroughness of Dr. Whitaker, we decided to go ahead with the program.

I must admit that the impact of the daily routine and diet was impressive. A great deal of thought and planning went into all the meals, but it still was quite different from our normal fare, as both of us cook as a hobby and belong to several gourmet clubs. Dr. Whitaker ate with us at all the meals and discussed various effects of the diet and exercise programs. He also supervised all exercise and constantly checked all the participants and several times requested that I rest for a while.

The first day I was barely able to slowly walk half a mile at any one session. At the end of the first week I could walk two miles at a fairly brisk pace. Also, the angina attacks became less frequent and much less severe. The daily lectures were extremely informative and made our effort more understanding. A closeness developed in our group, and we constantly encouraged and applauded each other's achievements. By the beginning of the second week the change in our life-styles was much easier to accept, and the marked improvement of everyone spurred us on.

By now I was walking four miles a day and the angina attacks had practically ceased. My amount of medication for my high blood pressure was cut in half and my weight had declined by two pounds. It may seem hard to comprehend, but at the completion of the program, none of us were in a hurry to leave.

Upon returning home, I continued with the diet and exercise programs. My original weight was 217, and after the first month home, it was below 190, on a six foot two inch frame. The angina had disappeared and I returned to a light routine of business activity and, at present, I am able to do most anything necessary for a complete life.

A year and a half later I returned to the Institute for a refresher course of five days. Dr. Whitaker had kept in touch every month or so by phone, and I informed him of all my involvements. He suggested a complete examination. I returned to Huntington Beach and learned some of the new therapy the doctor was using and had a thallium scan performed at the Hoag Hospital at Newport Beach. The results were amazing. My heart was completely normal.

At present I am in the process of building a room to install a small gym. Next month will be two years since my first visit to Dr. Whitaker.

The purpose of this account is to attempt to inform others of the benefits I have derived from this program and to thank Dr. Whitaker for the improvement in the quality of my life.

Case History

Lester Mendelsohn *Castro Valley, California*

I am sixty-nine years old. In March 1975, I had a stroke that seriously affected my left arm and leg. In October 1979, I had an angina attack. An angiogram was taken in January 1980. The diagnosis was that I needed four bypasses; but being considered a poor operative risk because of the stroke and hardening of the arteries, surgery was not performed, but I have been on medication.

In June 1980, I had trouble breathing. My wife took me to a local emergency hospital; my heartbeat was very irregular and very slow. It was arranged for me to see a doctor the following Monday, and in the meantime, the heart specialist prescribed a medication to regulate the heartbeat.

After the doctor completed the examination he told me that in view of the severe case of hardening of the arteries, nothing could be done for me except to continue the medication. This left my wife and myself depressed but determined that we would look for an alternative. My daughter mentioned having heard Dr. Whitaker on station KGO, and both she and my wife felt that we should contact him. My wife called the following day and spoke with Dr. Whitaker, who was very encouraging and was certain that his program of diet and exercise could help me.

I was a patient in his Institute for twelve days. I was immediately started on a program of nutrition and exercise. My exercise program consisted of pedaling a stationary bike for thirty minutes twice a day. I was also given vitamin supplements three times a day.

Results from the first to last blood test showed much improvement in my cholesterol level, as well as my triglycerides. Now, four months later, I am still following the diet and exercise plan. My heartbeat is regular, stronger, and not as slow. I have lost ten pounds. I look and feel better. I have eliminated some medications and cut down on others.

I am certainly happy that instead of giving up I went to Dr. Whitaker.

Case History

Donna Monroe *Buhl, Idaho*

I have been a patient of Dr. Julian Whitaker's and would like to express my gratitude and thanks to the National Heart and Diabetes Treatment Institute.

In December 1978, I had open heart surgery. However, after three or four months, I again experienced angina and never fully felt like the surgery did me much good. I continued to go downhill and experienced the same symptoms as before surgery. Finally, my cardiologist suggested that I have surgery again. This I refused, and with the help of my daughter in California, and friends who had heard of Dr. Whitaker, I decided I had nothing to lose by attending the Institute.

My husband and I entered the Institute in mid-April of 1980. Within one week, my blood pressure had dropped considerably. I experienced less angina and also my cholesterol drop was amazing. At the time of my surgery, I weighed 130 pounds at five feet one inch tall. At present I weigh exactly 100 pounds, and my blood pressure has stabilized to a safe and unbelievable level. As a grandmother of seven and a mother of three children, I now feel this life is once again worthwhile. I am no longer taking high blood pressure medication that I had taken for thirty-two years. I exercise and try to keep on my diet. I feel that Dr. Whitaker and his methods are much more helpful and encouraging than surgery. At least I now know that I never would go though that surgery again. If I do have problems, I know what I am doing wrong and can correct them.

Case History

William Wolf *Ithaca, New York*

I'm writing to share my experience at the National Heart and Diabetes Treatment Institute. I had a heart attack and had gone through the University of Washington Hospital, where I had been diagnosed as having approximately 20 percent damage to my left ventricle and two blocked arteries. My left anterior descending artery was 100 percent blocked, and the doctors were very forceful in advising that I have bypass surgery. Instead, I elected to follow a medical program. The statistics I was able to find indicated that bypass surgery would reduce pain but would not increase longevity. In addition, I was aware that there were a number of hazards or risks in bypass surgery. For example, when one is on the heart-lung machine, there tends to be a direct correlation between the length of time on the machine and strokes. There is also the question as to whether or not the operation itself causes heart attacks, etc. Consequently, I was very disturbed by the prescription of bypass surgery. I had a negative reaction to the angiogram and was placed in intensive care at the University of Washington Hospital. While in intensive care, one of the nurses reinforced my belief that I should seek a medical solution first. She advised me against rushing into an operation while I was in an upset state and suggested that I first try the Pritikin program. She was so positive about the program that when I got out of the hospital, I immediately bought Pritikin's book and tried to follow the program on my own. I must say that, although I read the book about seven times, I did not seem to make complete progress. I was still having pain. When I tried to exercise or walk, I frequently just had to stop to sit down and rest. I could not keep going. Thus, I was distraught and thought that I would have to go in for bypass surgery.

By chance, I met Don Kennedy on the beach. He had been fighting the same problem and had given up and was planning to go in for a bypass. He disappeared from Laguna Beach for several weeks, and when I saw him again, he looked great. I asked him about his bypass operation. He informed me that rather than a bypass he had been at the National Heart and Diabetes Institute. Thus, I called and immediately tried to get into the Institute.

By the time I entered the Institute, I had lost about fifteen pounds.

I was doing fairly well, but my blood pressure was still a little high. My triglycerides were way up. They were around 238. My cholesterol, which was rather high, was 261. My HDL was also very low—about 30.

I began to improve immediately. By the end of two weeks I was able to go seven or eight miles without undue fatigue. I would walk and do a slow jog for that distance. I was having only very minor pains; those usually occurred when I was warming up. My vital signs improved significantly. After two weeks my cholesterol level was down to 154, my triglycerides were down to 90, and my HDL was now up to 94. In short, all the measures of risk for heart attack had improved significantly. I was amazed at the results. I have returned to work and have been doing relatively well. I find that I cannot, in this climate in New York, really do the walking and jogging. But I am able to swim approximately thirty-five to forty lengths of the swimming pool, and usually I walk and jog two to five miles every other day. In short, I find that I am able to function effectively even with the impaired circulatory system.

What impressed me most about the program was Dr. Whitaker's personality and the way in which we were educated and led by precept and example so that we could understand and develop proper life-styles. I left the Institute improved and with a great deal more hope and confidence about my health.

Case History

Joann Lang — *Palo Alto, California*

Because of "suspicious" chest pains in 1972, I had an angiogram and the bypass operation. I was frightened, and from that time on, I had considered myself a cardiac cripple. In 1979, I had a heart attack and a repeat angiogram, which showed that both the graft and the artery were completely closed.

I entered Dr. Whitaker's program to do something positive about this problem. Now I have no chest pain. I joyously walk two to three miles a day, feel fantastic, and no longer consider myself a cardiac cripple. I wish I had done this before surgery.

Case History

Carlo Teodori *Lawrence, Pennsylvania*

In May 1980, I was told by my doctor of nine years that he thought I should increase my medication for high blood pressure. Since I was already taking three pills a day, I didn't want to increase that dosage.

I read in *Prevention* magazine that Dr. Whitaker in California was having success in lowering blood pressure by proper diet and exercise. I called him and he encouraged me to enroll in the Institute and try the program. My wife and I arrived the next week and started right in on the food prepared especially for the patients at the Institute. The very next morning we were up and walking with the other patients. Within a few days Dr. Whitaker suggested that I reduce my medication under his careful supervision. By the end of our two-week stay, I was off all medication and walking eight to ten miles a day and feeling great.

Since leaving the Institute, I have only taken medication twice when my pressure started to go back up. I then called Dr. Whitaker and he suggested I go on a rice and fruit diet for a few days and be sure to exercise at least enough to sweat for half an hour a day. This is working for me and I am grateful for Dr. Whitaker and the approach he used to eliminate my high blood pressure problem.

Diary of a Patient

Dr. John Fisher *Los Angeles, California*

It happened! How in the world could it happen to me? I always had annual physicals, was on medication for hypertension, medication for two ulcers (duodenal and pyloric), medication for hiatal hernia. Lost weight, gained weight. Saw my doctor because of chest pains. Always a negative EKG. Stress tests, too, proved negative. Always in the normal range. Blood work always in the normal range. People told me I was a typical, classic Friedman's Type A. Doctor and friends always warned me to slow down—that I would have a heart attack. Tried to slow down. Took vitamins. I knew that I had to lose weight.

Well, October 3, 1979, found me at a large auditorium ready to address about 500 administrators. Before my presentation I developed chest pains. I dismissed this discomfort, thinking it was my ulcer acting up, but it was higher and more persistent. I fulfilled my responsibility, left the podium, and began to feel terrible. I asked my friend for some antacid (Mylanta pills), but this discomfort not only persisted but became harsher. I asked my friend to drive me to my car as soon as possible. My chest felt heavy—tight—pain in the center of my chest. Finally got to my car, feebly opened the door to get my liquid antacid, Riopan. No relief. Pain was severe. I was perspiring. I set out for the hospital. I found myself taking deep breaths and trying to find the right street. I felt disconnected, and fear began to creep into my mind. Finally I saw the hospital, parked the car, and walked into the admitting room. I must have looked frightened and terrible because I was quickly admitted and waited for the doctor. The doctor looked at me, listened to my heart, ordered an EKG, and informed me that I was having a heart attack. I was immediately wheeled to another room, given shots, and an IV was started. I became familiar with a new term (for me)—myocardial infarction.

I was admitted to intensive care. There was a natural fear and apprehension especially that first night when a patient was wheeled out of the ward because he had expired. I had a second attack about four or five days later because of straining from a bowel impaction. This was so painful and a great concern to nurses and doctor. I spent two weeks in the hospital on medication. I still awakened with chest discomfort, tightness, and heaviness.

I was sent home armed with literature, medication, and what I thought was a new way of life. I lost weight. I wanted to become healthy. I read American Heart Association literature, books, and literature the hospital gave me about heart disease, and Norman Cousins's book for attitude. And so the recuperative period started. Followed the doctor's instructions to the letter. Angina persisted at home. The doctor ordered me back to the hospital. I rested a few days. It was decided that I should have an angiogram. Yes, there was a blockage, but the decision to do a bypass was negative. I was relieved and pleased. No surgery—I didn't want that to happen. Returned home again and participated in a heart rehabilitation program at another hospital. This consisted of monitored exercise, relaxation, and biofeedback. Finally I felt like going back to work. I was determined to go back to work and rescue my life.

I was on the following medications:

Inderal	60 mg	4 × a day
Isordil	5 mg	4 × a day
Surfak	240 mg	2 × a day (stool softener)
Hydrodiural		
KCL		A.M. and P.M.

Valium, as needed (I never took these because of the bad publicity.)
Antacid—Mylanta II

Got back on the administrative merry-go-round. I visited my doctor every six weeks. I decided diet was important after reading Pritikin's book. I took a course that highlighted the Pritikin diet. I began to eat what I thought was sensible. I gained weight, and my blood work indicated an elevation of cholesterol and triglycerides. Still had angina, which frightened and concerned me. Why, why did this persist? Was I causing it? Was it all in my head? Took a treadmill test. Negative, everything okay. Then why did I get angina when I walked? Time passed—still uneasy. Triglycerides went from 200 to 300, 400, 500, 600. Called my doctor. Had some more blood work done. The doctor then prescribed Atromid S.

I wasn't feeling well. My weight went up to 190, then down to 183. Felt poorly physically and was feeling despondent. I experienced impotency. I was not myself. Felt poorly emotionally—increased fatigue, shortness of breath, and, most of all, fear. I was frustrated, disappointed, and most unhappy.

The next thing that happened to me was like a miracle. I hesitate to tell it because it sounds so make-believe.

I have always slept poorly, therefore I keep a radio on most of the night listening to KABC. This night I awakened to hear someone saying (and I paraphrase), "If anyone is on Atromid S, they ought to get off it as it is a poor drug, can be fatal in some cases, and it has been banned in Europe." I got up and listened. The person speaking was a Dr. Whitaker. I listened the rest of the morning. Took his phone number and address. He seemed to make so much sense.

The next day I called my doctor and told him I no longer wanted to take Atromid S because I thought it was causing my impotency. He told me that if it was that important to me, to stop taking the drug. I made other observations that concerned me. My fingernails felt bumpy. I experienced a loss of hair from my head. I felt lousy.

I had to do something. I needed a second opinion. I called Dr. Whitaker's office and requested an appointment. I received literature describing his twelve-day program. I was skeptical because of the cost of the program. Remember, I was most distrustful of doctors because of what was happening to me. I wasn't getting any help and I wasn't getting better.

I found myself at five o'clock in the morning heading for Huntington Beach and Dr. Whitaker's office. I planned to get there early to look around and talk to patients and generally see for myself what was going on. I drove to a motel beautifully situated across the street from the Pacific Ocean. The air smelled good. The Huntington Beach Inn is attractive, with a golf course in back. Generally impressed, but what was a doctor doing here? I inquired at the reception desk where the National Heart and Diabetes Treatment Institute was located. I was told room 120. Walked to room 120, which appeared to be another room in the motel. Walked back to my car and drove it close to the room. Waited until 8:00 A.M., when it opened. It was a doctor's reception room. Men and women were entering. I went in and talked to some of these people—asked questions. I learned that they were patients. They talked about themselves. Their general outlook was positive. I was favorably impressed.

My appointment with Dr. Whitaker was at 9:00 A.M. I met a young man who appeared interested in my problems. He listened to me and gave me frank answers. He appeared to be a person in whom I wanted to believe. I gave him my background. No, he would not accept me as an outpatient. It would be wise if I could participate in the twelve-day program at a cost of $2,800. This was a lot of money for me as I was not employed during the summer. I told him about my radio experience and Atromid S and that I had discontinued it after hearing his broadcast. I left his office in an ambivalent state. Why would a doctor set up in a motel? Yes, I was impressed with the doctor. I was impressed after listening to his patients. I had to do something. I didn't feel I was getting better. I felt that I had to grab what I considered to be the last straw.

Returned home and told my wife that I would enter the Institute. I made arrangements with my superiors and also borrowed the money so that I could participate. The program is set up so that the patient and a partner attend together, which impressed me. I went alone because of family obligations. My wife had to help our son and daughter-in-law with the care of twins. After returning from San

Francisco she had to help our daughter care for a newborn baby girl. So I left home and returned to participate in Dr. Whitaker's program. I arrived on Sunday, checked in at the reception desk, got my room, and unpacked. At 3:15 P.M. my phone rang. It was Dr. Whitaker, who asked me to come down for a physical at 4:00 P.M.

I brought copies of my lab reports and a list of all the supplements I was taking in addition to the drugs that were prescribed for me. Dr. Whitaker asked about my heart attack. He read the reports from the hospital. He stated that we would cut my medication gradually and introduce niacin and one hour of breathing oxygen. He examined my eyes, listened to my chest, and palpated my stomach. This took about thirty minutes. He bid me good-bye and said that he would see me at dinner at 5:30 P.M. He kept the lab reports and the list of supplements and medicines.

I went away encouraged. I had been asking my doctor in Los Angeles to lower the amount of medication. He always put me off and said I needed it. I returned to my room with my vitamins and other information I shared with Dr. Whitaker. This was the first time I ever shared the information on the supplements I was taking. Dr. Whitaker suggested I cut out the zinc because there was enough in the other combinations. My point is that I was going to be direct and honest with the doctor as I wanted him to know exactly what I was taking. The other doctors "pooh-poohed" the supplements. I was here to get well—to get another opinion—to do everything with determination and effort. Dr. Whitaker's attitude, friendliness, and down-to-business nature invited my reaction.

Well, I went to dinner. Introductions were made. Dr. Whitaker was there, and you know what? He sat down and ate exactly what we ate. As time went on we became a close-knit group—caring for one another and praising our accomplishments. We encouraged one another, and each of us had a sense of pride for each other's accomplishments. But, I'm getting ahead of myself. I must tell you about our first meal. I remember it because I kept a diary while I was at the Institute. This was to help me remember so that I could evaluate my progress and help to plan my future. Our first dinner together was the beginning of twelve days of eating, exercising, relaxing, and taking oxygen together. Our first meal was served attractively. The table was always carefully set. We had and, may I add, enjoyed a salad consisting of lettuce, carrots, and peas with a dressing that contained no oil. On the table at every meal we had raisins. We were told to eat two teaspoons at every meal. We also had a packet of vitamins and niacin. We were then served a good portion of whole-wheat spaghetti in a most delicious sauce with sapsago cheese. It was delicious. The dinner ended with fruit. We had a choice of Sanka or herb tea. Apple butter was on the table as a spread for bread or pancakes. We were invited to take some fruit for a midnight snack. This was the beginning of many pleasant meals. The genuine friendliness of all enhanced each meal—but our leader, our doctor, set the tone—good sense of humor, keen interest in all of us, answered questions directly, kept his promises, and was sincere.

I walked back to my room after dinner as I would for the ensuing duration of my stay, to lay out my clothes for the next day, to write in my diary, to read for a while, and then to sleep.

The next day I awakened early, 4:30 A.M., went for a walk, came back, showered, and got ready to follow the daily schedule we received at our orientation. We reported to the office each day to weigh in and take our blood pressure. On this day my weight was 181½ pounds, my blood pressure was 125/80, and my pulse was also taken. We then went to breakfast, which consisted of orange juice, three buckwheat hotcakes, Butter Buds for topping, honey, which was always available, herb tea, and vitamins. I began with 100 mg niacin. Everything was so delicious and served with such pride. After breakfast we were to report to the doctor's office for an EKG and stress test. After the test Dr. Whitaker explained that I did well on the EKG and then wrote out my exercise prescription. I was to walk briskly one mile in the morning and two miles in the afternoon. I was to get my pulse up to between 90 and 110. Dr. Whitaker also said I was overmedicated. He said we were going to lower the amount of medication. He reduced Inderal that first day from 60 mg four times per day to 60 mg three times per day. This medication was lowered gradually until at the end of my stay I was taking only 20 mg of Inderal per day. I would also inhale oxygen one hour per day. I found I could do this by inhaling for thirty minutes after breakfast and thirty minutes after morning exercise. I am still on oxygen inhalation. Because of my work I have changed my oxygen schedule to thirty minutes when I return home from work and thirty minutes after dinner.

After our EKG testing we all met with the doctor at 10:00 A.M. for our exercise session. I walked twice around a three-quarter-mile track. Pulse was close to 90. Dr. Whitaker was with us, taking our pulse, advising us, reviewing and giving us personal attention. This was so important. His encouragement and concern were genuine and meant a lot to me. Dr. Whitaker was always there during the exercise period.

After our exercise period I went to inhale oxygen again, then to shower and change clothing. Before we knew it, it was lunchtime. Not only did the doctor come to lunch with us, but the nurse and receptionist ate with us as well. For our lunch the first day we had a portion of rice with steamed vegetables consisting of cauliflower and squash. Salad, a large baked potato, and small slices of pineapple rounded out the lunch. All this was served on a large platter. There were oohs and aahs because of the amount of food and the size of the platter. It was colorful and appetizing.

After lunch we attended a lecture. Dr. Whitaker would lecture on a different subject each day with a slide presentation. Each lecture provided and cited studies from medical journals, periodicals, and newspaper articles. I looked forward to these educational sessions. These seminars provided understanding, new information, clarification, and reasons for doing and following the regimen.

After the lectures we prepared ourselves for our afternoon exercise. We would do this independently or in small groups. When we completed our exercise period we would prepare for our relaxation session. First, we would lie down on mats. Dr. Whitaker would then direct our relaxation to various parts of our body. This led to total body relaxation and was accomplished while listening to pleasant music. A few patients would relax to the point of sleep. After this period we would ready ourselves for dinner at 5:30 P.M.

Guess who came to dinner? You're right! Our doctor was there to dine with us, converse, answer questions, and advise. Because of his pleasing, positive attitude he made his patients care about this new regimen. For dinner the first day we ate a tomato-lettuce salad, a bowl of chili, two slices of wheat bread, a slice of melon, and herb tea. At each meal we had our packet of vitamins, niacin, and any other medication we were taking. There was a large bowl of fruit. We were invited to help ourselves so that we could have a snack before sleep. I walked back to my room, got my clothes ready, watched TV, read, and I was ready for bed. Tired but a good tiredness.

The food at the Institute was prepared deliciously. I learned I could eat vegetables, grains, and fruits. We enjoyed it because it was prepared simply and beautifully.

My progress was dramatic. Every day I weighed myself. By the time I was ready to leave I had dropped from 181½ to 176. That was great, but let me tell you how excited I was to have my blood pressure taken and find out I was 120/78 with less medication. The lab work was really thrilling. Remember, I had a triglyceride of 309, 225 of cholesterol, and 24 HDL. The second report read 109 triglyceride, 186 cholesterol. It was dramatic. Just before we left we had blood work done again. Dr. Whitaker called me at home to tell me the results of the last lab report—triglycerides 100, cholesterol 157, and HDL 39. Excellent. I was thrilled. Imagine, my doctor called me to tell me of the progress I had made. This was great. I feel I am on my way to better health. I'm going to reverse my condition with my new dedication to better health. No one can realize how thrilled and excited I am. I am losing weight. I am eating less and better. My attitude toward life is a lot better. I have less fear. I am not depressed. I am not experiencing impotency the way I was. My nails seem to be healthier. My pulse when walking is averaging 114 to 120 and sometimes 126. What progress. Yes, I am still bothered by some angina, but I feel so much better. My friends and family tell me how much better I look and how much calmer I seem. "What have you done?" they ask me. This is so encouraging. I feel great.

From the Alumni

Homer G. Ray *Atlanta, Georgia*

The two weeks my wife and I spent at the National Heart and Diabetes Treatment Institute, early in 1980, were undoubtedly one of the finest things we have done for our health and well-being in many years. The time and energy consumed and the expense of travel from Atlanta to California were worthwhile. We have unhesitatingly recommended the Institute to friends here in Georgia. Those two weeks brought about changes in our life-styles and eating habits that are continuing and benefiting us.

The good attention that Dr. Whitaker gave us, and the fellowship with others then in attendance, made it a most stimulating and enjoyable two weeks. I am now considering making it an annual event in our lives because of the benefits and enrichment that it brought to us. Some of us are careless in our eating and living habits in day-to-day living, and what Dr. Whitaker offers in direction and supervision is most helpful in bringing about good changes in lifestyle and diet. I think we would all be far better off if we would take at least two weeks a year and, in the spirit of Dr. Whitaker's program, give our health needs the top priority.

Otto Lauf *Scottsdale, Arizona*

I would like to take this opportunity to join the thousands of others who have shared the experience of attending Dr. Julian Whitaker's National Heart and Diabetes Treatment Institute.

In 1979, I suffered a total collapse and was told that I would be facing open heart surgery. My cholesterol level was so high, it seemed like the only solution if I wanted to live a normal life. It was not a prospect that I looked forward to, and I immediately began looking for an alternative solution. It was then that I heard about attending Dr. Whitaker's Institute.

I attended a two-week session and found the only thing I had in my favor was my weight. I had never had a weight problem. My eating habits and way of life were decreasing my longevity.

Through Dr. Whitaker's program of diet and exercise, a whole new life has opened up to me. I've learned to eat properly and, though I sometimes yearn for a thick, juicy steak, I find that following his diet can be an enjoyable experience.

My cholesterol level has dropped drastically. Each checkup has shown very marked improvement. I walk three miles every morning, have played thirty-six holes of golf in one day, and have not been sick in over a year. I have a whole new attitude toward my health and life, feel years younger, and I am enjoying things that I never thought were possible.

My thanks to Dr. Whitaker and his staff, who, through their care and guidance, have given me a new lease on life.

Joseph Moriconi *Manchester, Connecticut*

I spent twelve days at Dr. Whitaker's Heart Institute with my wife. It was the best money I have ever spent for my health. My cholesterol level dropped from 223 to 184. I stopped using Inderal. My blood pressure stays steady at 120/80. I have 90 percent heart blockage of my two main arteries. The blockage is in a place where the bypass operation is risky. I know that if I continue to follow the program I went through at Dr. Whitaker's, which I will, I will be able to live a good normal life.

Mildred Jessup *Laguna Hills, California*

I think of Dr. Whitaker with appreciation for the way he changed my life. I went to him because I was sick—I had always had a weight problem and arthritis. I felt I had to do something to give my body all the help I could so I could feel good at my age. I also wanted to do what I could to avoid other degenerative problems, such as heart attack, stroke, diabetes, etc.

In going through his program, I learned the relationship of foods to the different organs of the body and also the damage that the wrong things can do. I lost fifteen pounds, but what is most important is that the weight has stayed off for over a year now. My arthritis has improved and I expect it to keep improving. My cholesterol and blood pressure both dropped. I have grown to love the taste of foods in their natural forms and do not find the fatty foods, red meat, and sweet junk palatable anymore.

Grace Mohler *Mission Viejo, California*

I am willing to tell everyone the excellent results I have had since I attended Dr. Whitaker's two-week program at the National Heart and Diabetes Institute. My cholesterol dropped from 325 to 216 in these two weeks and has stayed low since, without medication. My blood pressure has also maintained a healthy level with less medication. I had never eaten so much, yet I still lost twenty pounds. This all sums up to a better attitude and a happier life. I still walk two to five miles a day. Indigestion, which I frequently had, is no more. I feel just great.

I started on this way of life in January 1980. I don't believe I could have accomplished all this from books. They are so well informed at the Institute, and this helped me to understand the whys and ways of eating and exercise.

Robert Clifford *Portola Valley, California*

In June of 1979, I had an abnormal treadmill test and underwent an angiogram. Even though I did not have chest pain or angina, I was advised to have the bypass operation. I enrolled in the National Heart and Diabetes Institute the day before I was to have surgery.

Now my cholesterol and triglycerides are very low. I've lost twenty-seven pounds in eight weeks, I am walking two miles a day with no pain. I feel great and plan to stay on this program and avoid surgery.

Dale Harris *Liberty, Missouri*

If I had known about this program earlier, I could have avoided a lot of grief and surgery. By the time I was fifty-four, I had already had the large artery in my stomach replaced with a plastic graft as well as the bypass operation on my heart for clogged arteries. In spite of this surgery, I still could not walk because of severe pain in my calves, due to the blockages in the other arteries as well as blockages coming on in the graft. It was time I did something, so I spent two weeks at the National Heart and Diabetes Treatment Institute in March of 1979. I learned how to eat, how to exercise, the role of vitamins and minerals, and just, in general, how to take care of myself.

I was amazed at how rapidly changes occur on this program. As a result of the life-style, the artery damage that I had suffered because of our rich diet surely slows down, stops, and hopefully reverses. I had always had a cholesterol problem and was even taking Atromid S for it without success. This problem was eliminated completely in just two weeks on the diet and a small dose of niacin. Other studies improved dramatically as well.

	Initial	Ending
Cholesterol	324(with Atromid)	130(with diet plan)
Triglycerides	413	123
Blood pressure	130/78	108/66

Exactly three years after leaving the Institute, I am happy to report that I am completely pain-free in my legs and have been so for the last two and one-half years. I am walking two miles every day and without any pain at all, feeling great and doing anything that I want to do. What a joy it is to be pain-free and getting healthy.

Ray and Ad Kimball *Littleton, Colorado*

June 6, 1984

Even though I was taking 130 units of insulin and seventeen prescription pills every day of my life, I was surprised to be at the Whitaker Clinic. After reading about Dr. Whitaker and the Institute in *Prevention* magazine, my wife had recommended we go. For the past two years she had literally begged me to go.

But I was not easily persuaded. As a "workaholic" who can't remember missing a day's work in the last thirty-five years, except for a one-night stay in the hospital after the removal of a "melanoma" mole, I wanted to try everything else first. And I did!

When I was diagnosed as "early onset diabetes," my personal reaction was perhaps typical. Trying to forestall the thought of the traditional insulin, I ran the gamut on Orinase and Diabanese. I even cheated by taking more than the doctor prescribed, hoping to avoid the needle. But the blood sugar levels kept rising, so I finally gave in and started on a modest level of insulin injections.

For nine months I had dutifully gone to the hospital twice a week for two blood tests. These automatically resulted in an increase of insulin intake until I reached the 130-units-per-day mark. In answer to my question, "Will this situation ever be better?" the doctor just flatly told me "No."

At this time I was also taking medication for high blood pressure and atrial fibrillation, resulting in the daily intake of the seventeen prescription pills daily.

While I'm grateful for the limited number of doctors who have literally saved my life in specific situations—Dr. Whitaker tops that list—I've surely had my share of medical kiss-offs of the "keep taking your present medications and call me if you need help" type!

When I finally arrived at the Whitaker Clinic in Huntington Beach, I was taking 130 units of insulin per day (44 of humulin R and 86 of humulin NPH) for diabetes, 2 hydrochlorothiazide, 8 "micro K" potassium pills, and 2 Midamor (another diuretic) for high blood pressure, plus 1 digoxin and 4 verapamil tablets for atrial fibrillation control.

Diet had hardly been mentioned all during this build-up of my "pathological museum." We had been told to use salt sparingly, and we cut out all sugar, thinking it was the culprit.

What a shocker we received at the Whitaker Institute. Dr. Whitaker placed me on a nonfat diet, and increased my exercise schedule. In two days I was totally "off insulin," and within a week I had discontinued all prescription pills. My blood sugar levels were, for the very first time in years, safely within the desired range of 80–120, my blood pressure remained at the same, or lower, levels I had achieved under medication, and my pulse was normal. At the end of the first week I had dropped six pounds. I really was a new person!

The clinic's nonfat diet, prepared personally by a registered nurse/professional nutritionist, was simple, adequate, and, best of all, understandable. Taking time to exercise was a scheduled luxury, and a totally new life-style was formulated—health, attitude, and commitment being the keys.

We will be forever grateful for the Whitaker Institute and the wonderful people associated with it.

BIBLIOGRAPHY

Suggested Recipe Books

Bond, Harry C. *Natural Food Cookbook.* North Hollywood, California: Wilshire Book Co., 1980.

Cadwallader, Sharon and Judi Ohr. *Whole Earth Cookbook.* New York: Bantam Books, 1973.

Campbell, Diane. *Step-by-Step to Natural Food.* Clearwater, Florida: Cancer Book House, 1981.

Connor, William, et al. *The Alternative Diet Book.* Iowa City, Iowa: University of Iowa Publications, 1976.

Eshleman, Ruthe and Mary Winston. *The American Heart Association Cookbook.* New York: David McKay, Inc., 1973.

Ewald, Ellen B. *Recipes for a Small Planet.* New York: Ballantine Books, 1975.

Ford, Frank. *The Simpler Life Cookbook: From Arrowhead Mills.* Waco, Texas: Hanest Press, 1974.

Gibbons, Barbara, and the editors of *Consumer Guide. Lean Cuisine.* Skokie, Illinois: Publications International, 1979.

Lappé, Frances Moore. *Diet for a Small Planet.* New York: Ballantine Books, 1970.

Leonard, Jon and Elaine Taylor. *The Live Longer Now Cookbook.* New York: Grosset and Dunlap, 1977.

Leviton, Roberta. *The Jewish Low-Cholesterol Cookbook.* Middlebury, Vermont: Erikkson Press, 1978.

Lo, Kenneth H. C. *Chinese Vegetarian Cookery.* New York: Pantheon Books, 1974.

Margie, Joyce and James Hunt. *Living with High Blood Pressure.* Bloomfield, New Jersey: HLS Press, 1978.

Martin, Faye. *Rodale's Naturally Delicious Desserts and Snacks.* Emmaus, Pennsylvania: Rodale Press, 1978.

Pritikin, Nathan. *The Pritikin Program for Diet and Exercise.* New York: Bantam Books, 1980.

Richmond, Sonya. *International Vegetarian Cookery.* New York: Arco Publishing Co., 1965.

Robertson, Laurel, Carol Flinders, and Bronwen Godfrey. *Laurel's Kitchen.* New York: Bantam Books, 1978.

Stern, Ellen and Jonathan Michaels. *The Good Heart Diet Cookbook.* New York: Warner Books, 1983.

Sunset Books. *Ideas for Cooking Vegetables.* Menlo Park, California: Lane Publishing Co., 1979.

Thomas, Anna. *The Vegetarian Epicure.* New York: Vintage, 1972.

Selected References

Åberg, Torkel, M.D. Effect of open heart surgery on intellectual function. *Scandinavian Journal of Thoracic and Cardiovascular Surgery.* Supplement 15, 1974.

——— et al. Release of adenylate kinase into cerebral spinal fluid during open heart surgery and its relation to post-operative intellectual function. *The Lancet.* 1139–1141, May 22, 1982.

Abraham, S. A., M.D. Effect of chromium on established atherosclerotic plaques in rabbits. *American Journal of Clinical Nutrition.* 33, 2294–2298, Nov. 1980.

Achuff, S. C., M.D. The angina producing myocardial segment, an approach to the interpretation of the results of coronary bypass surgery. *American Journal of Cardiology.* 36: 723, 1975.

Alfin-Slater, Rosylyn, M.D. Plasma cholesterol in triglycerides in men with added eggs in the diet. *Nutrition Reports International.* Vol. 14: 249–259, 1976.

Angina after bypass surgery: Specialist explains why pain recurs in so many patients. *Acute Care Medicine.* 33–50: Feb. 1984.

Anitschkow, N. Über experimentelle Cholesterin Steatose und ihre Bedeutung fur die Entstehung einiger pathologischer. *Prozesse: Zbl. Path.* 26: 1, 1913.

Armstrong, Mark L., M.D. Progression of coronary atheromatosis in rhesus monkeys. *Circulation Research.* 27: 59–67, 1970.

———. Arterial fibrous proteins and cynomolgus monkeys after atherogenic and regression diets. *Circulation Research.* 36: 256–261, 1975.

Ashoff, T., M.D. Lectures in pathology. New York: Hoeber, 1924.

Barash, Paul, G., M.D. Cardiopulmonary bypass and post-operative neurologic dysfunction. *American Heart Journal.* 99: 675–677, 1980.

Barndt, R., Jr., M.D. and D. H. Blankenhorn, M.D. Regression and progression of early femoral atherosclerosis in treated hyperlipoproteinemic patients. *Annals of Internal Medicine.* 86: 139–143, 1977.

Bassler, T., M.D. Regression of athroma. *Western Journal of Medicine.* 132: 474–75, 1980.

Basta, L. L., M.D. Regression of atherosclerotic stenosing lesions of the renal arteries and spontaneous cure of systemic hypertension through control of hyperlipidemia. *American Journal of Medicine.* 61: 420–423, 1976.

Bayoumi, R. A., M.D. and S. B. Rosalki, M.D. Evaluation of methods of coenzyme activation of erythrocyten enzymes of detection of deficiency of Vitamins B_1, B_2, B_6. *Clinical Chemistry.* 22: 327, 1976.

Beecher, H. K., M.D. Surgery as placebo: A quantitative study of bias. *Journal of the American Medical Association.* 176: 1102, 1961.

Belizan, J. M., M.D. Reduction of blood pressure with calcium supplementation in young adults. *Journal of the American Medical Association.* 249: 1161–1165, 1983.

Beveridge, J. M. R., M.D. The response of man to dietary cholesterol. *Journal of Nutrition.* 71: 61, 1960.

Bourassa, M. G., M.D. Changes in grafts in coronary arteries after saphenous vein aortic coronary bypass surgery, results at repeat angiography. *Circulation.* 65 (Part 2): II, 90–7, 1982.

———. Progression of coronary arterial disease after coronary artery bypass grafts. *Circulation.* 47 (Supplement 3): 111, 127, 1973.

Brain damage after open heart surgery, an editorial. *The Lancet.* 1161–1163, May 22, 1982.

Braunwald, E., M.D. Coronary artery bypass surgery, an assessment. *Post-graduate Medical Journal.* 52: 733, 1976.

———. Coronary artery surgery at the crossroads. An editorial. *New England Journal of Medicine.* 297: 661–663, 1977.

———. Editorial retrospective, effects of coronary artery bypass grafting on survival; implications of the randomized coronary artery surgery study. *New England Journal of Medicine.* 309, 1181–1184, Nov. 1983.

Buccino, Robert A., M.D. Aorto-coronary bypass grafting in patients with coronary artery disease. *Primary Cardiology.* 91–95, Jan. 1981.

Campeau, L., M.D. Loss of the improvement of angina between 1 and 7 years after aorta coronary bypass surgery: Correlations with changes in vein grafts and in coronary arteries. *Circulation.* 60 (Supplement I): I, 1–5, 1979.

Cashin, W. Linda, M.D., et al. Accelerated progression of atherosclerosis in coronary vessels with minimal lesions that are bypassed. *New England Journal of Medicine.* 311: 824–828, 1984.

Chenoweth, Dennis E., Ph.D. Complement activation during cardiopulmonary bypass. *New England Journal of Medicine.* 304: 497–503, 1981.

———. Complement activation during cardiopulmonary bypass: Evidence for generation of C3A and C5A ahaphylatoxins. *New England Journal of Medicine.* 304: 497–503, 1981.

Chesebro, James H., M.D. Effect of dipyridamole and aspirin on late vein-graft patency after coronary bypass operations. *New England Journal of Medicine.* 310: 209–214, 1984.

Cobb, Leonard A., M.D. An evaluation of internal mammary artery ligation by doubleblind technique. *New England Journal of Medicine.* 260: 1115–1118, 1959.

Connor, W. E., M.D. Serum lipids in men receiving high cholesterol and cholesterol-free diets. *Journal of Clinical Investigation.* 40: 894, 1961.

Cornfeld, D. S., M.D. Delirium after coronary bypass surgery. *The Journal of Thoracic and Cardiovascular Surgery.* 76: 93–96, 1978.

Coronary Artery Surgery Study (CASS). Myocardial infarction and mortality in the CASS randomized trial. *New England Journal of Medicine.* 310: 750–758, 1984.

Coronary Artery Surgery Study (CASS). A randomized trial of coronary artery bypass surgery, quality of life in patients randomly assigned to treatment groups. *Circulation.* 68: 951–960, 1983.

Coronary Artery Surgery Study (CASS). A randomized trial of coronary artery bypass surgery, survival data. *Circulation.* 68: 939–950, 1983.

Dimond, E. Grey, M.D. Comparison on internal mammary ligation and sham operation for angina pectoris. *American Journal of Cardiology.* 5: 483–486, 1960.

Elwood, J. C., Ph.D. Effect of high chromium brewers yeast on human serum lipids. *Journal of American College of Nutrition.* 1: 263–274, 1982.

Finamore, F. J., M.D. L-Ascorbic Acid, L-Ascorbate, 2-Sulfate and Atherogenesis. *International Journal of Vitamins and Nutrition Research.* 46:275–285, 1976.

Fitzgibbon, G. M., M.D. Coronary bypass graft fate: angiographic grading of 1400 consecutive grafts early after operation and of 1132 after one year. *Circulation.* 57, 1070–1074, 1978.

Flynn, Margaret A., Ph.D. Effective dietary egg on human serum cholesterol and triglycerides. *American Journal of Clinical Nutrition.* 32: 1051–1057, 1979.

Freis, E. D., M.D. Should mild hypertension be treated? *New England Journal of Medicine.* 307: 306–9, 1982.

Friedman, G. D., M.D. Decline in hospitalization for coronary heart disease and stroke: the Kaiser-Permanente experience in northern California, 1971–1977. In: Havlik, R., Feinleib, eds., *Proceedings of the Conference on the Decline of Coronary Heart Disease Mortality, Bethesda, October 24–25, 1978.* U.S. Department of Health, Education and Welfare. DHEW Report No. (NIH) 79-1610, pages 109–114, 1979.

Friedman, Meyer, M.D. *Type A Behavior and Your Heart.* New York: Alfred A. Knopf, 1974.

Ginter, E., M.D. The role of ascorbic acid in cholesterol catabolism and atherogenesis. Slovak Academy of Sciences, Bratislava. 1975.

Goodnight, Scott, H., M.D. and Dr. W. E. Connor, M.D. The effects of dietary ω3 fatty acids on platelet composition and function in man: A perspective control study. *Journal of Blood.* 58: 880–885, 1981.

Greist, John H., M.D. Antidepressant running, running as a treatment for non-psychotic depression. *Behavioral Medicine.* July 19, 1979.

Griffin, J. C., M.D. Recurring angina in patients following coronary bypass surgery. *Practical Cardiology.* 57–64, Dec. 1978.

Griffith, L. S. C., M.D. Changes in intrinsic coronary circulation and segmental vetricular motion after saphenous vein coronary bypass graft surgery. *New England Journal of Medicine.* 288: 589, 1973.

Grimm, Richard H., Jr., M.D. Effects of thiazide diuretics on plasma lipids and lipoproteins in mildly hypertensive patients. *Annals of Internal Medicine.* 94: 7–11, 1981.

Haeger, Knut, M.D. Long term treatment of intermittent claudication with vitamin E. *The American Journal of Clinical Nutrition.* 27:1179–1181, 1974.

———. The treatment of peripheral occlusive arterial disease with alpha tocopherol as compared with vasodilitator agents and antiprothrombin (Dicumarol). *Vascular Diseases.* 5: 199, 1968.

Harrell, Ruth, M.D. Can nutritional supplements help men with retarded children? An exploratory study and proceedings of the National Academy of Science, 78: 574–578, January, 1981.

Hegsted, D. M., M.D. Safe allowance of protein. *American Journal of Clinical Nutrition.* 29: 465, 1976.

Helgeland, Anders, M.D. Treatment of mild hypertension, a 5 year controlled drug trial, The Oslo Study. *American Journal of Medicine.* 69: 725–732, 1980.

Henriksen, Leif, M.D. Evidence suggestive of diffuse brain damage following cardiac operations. *The Lancet.* 816–820, April 14, 1984.

Herbert, V., M.D. Destruction of vitamin B_{12} by ascorbic acid. *Journal of the American Medical Association.* 230: 241–242, 1974.

———. The vitamin craze. *Archives of Internal Medicine.* 148:173, 1980.

Hermann, William J., Jr., M.D. The effect of tocopherol on high density lipoprotein cholesterol. *American Journal of Clinical Pathology.* 72: 848–852, 1979.

Higher death rates in hypertensive patients treated with diuretics raise many questions. *Cardiovascular News.* 12, Oct. 1984. (Discussions of Study by Dr. Gary Cutter.)

Hill, J. D., M.D. Neuropathological manifestations of cardiac surgery. *Annals of Thoracic Surgery.* 7: 409–419, 1969.

Holland, O. B., M.D. Diuretic induced ventricular ectopic activity. *American Journal of Medicine.* 70: 762–768, 1981.

Horrobin, David F., M.D., Editor. *Clinical uses of essential fatty acids.* Montreal, Canada: The Eden Press Inc., 1982.

Ignatowski, A. Über die Wirkung des tierischen Eiweisses auf die Aorta und die parkenchromatösen Organe der Kaninchen. *Virchos Arch.* 198: 248, 1909.

Imai, Hideshige. Angiotoxicity of oxygenated sterols and possible precursors. *Science.* 207: 651–653, 1980.

International Medical News Service. Decreased MI mortality: search for explanations. *Internal Medicine News.* 15: 1 no. 9, May 1–14, 1982. (Report of work by Dr. Sidney Pell.)

Johnson, Nancy E., M.D. Effect of level of protein intake on urinary and equal calcium, and calcium retention of young adult males. *Journal of Nutrition.* 100: 1425–1430, 1970.

Kannell, W. B., M.D., and W. P. Castelli, M.D. Serum cholesterol lipoproteins and risk of coronary heart disease, the Framingham study. *Annals of Internal Medicine.* 24: 1, 1971.

Kaplan, Norman, M.D. Current controversy: salt in hypertension. *Dateline Hypertension.* 2: 1, Jan. 1984.

Keys, Ancel, M.D. Lessons from serum cholesterol studies in Japan, Hawaii and Los Angeles. *Annals of Internal Medicine.* 48: 83, 1958.

———. Coronary heart disease in 7 countries. *American Heart Association Monograph.* 29. Also in *Circulation.* 41 (Supplement 1): 1970.

Kjeldsen, K., M.D., Reversal of rabbit atheromatosis by hyperoxia. *Journal of Atherosclerosis Research.* 10: 173–178, 1969.

Kothari, L. K., M.D. Effective vitamin C administration on blood cholesterol levels in man. *Act. Biologica,* Academy of Science, Hungary. 28, 111–114, 1977.

Kramsch, Dieter M. Reduction of coronary atherosclerosis by moderate conditioning exercise in monkeys on an atherogenic diet. *New England Journal of Medicine.* 305: 1483–1489, 1981.

Kuo, Peter T., M.D. Angina pectoris induced by fat ingestion in patients with coronary artery disease. *Journal of the American Medical Association.* 1008–1013, July 23, 1955.

Lee, K. T., M.D. Production of advanced coronary atherosclerosis, myocardial infarction and "sudden death" in swine. *Experimental Molecular Pathology.* 15: 170–190, 1971.

Leslie, Constance, M.D. Miracle that can lower cholesterol. *Family Circle.* 10–14, 1975.

Levy, Robert I., M.D. Declining mortality in coronary heart disease. *Arteriosclerosis.* 1: 312–325, Sept./Oct. 1981.

Logue, Bruce, M.D. A practical approach to coronary artery disease, with special reference to coronary artery bypass surgery. *Current Problems in Cardiology.* 1: 5, 1976.

Lonsdale, D., M.D., and R. J. Shamberger, M.D. Red cell transketolase as an indicator of nutritional deficiency. *American Journal of Clinical Nutrition.* 33: 205, 1980.

MacGregor, Graham A., Moderate potassium supplementation in essential hypertension. *The Lancet.* 567–570, Sept. 11, 1982.

Malmros, H., M.D. The relation of nutrition to health—A statistical study of the effect of wartime on atherosclerosis, cardiosclerosis, tuberculosis and diabetes. *Activ. Med. Scandinavia.* Supplement 246: 137–153, 1950.

Mann, George G., M.D. Cardiovascular disease in the Masai. *Journal Atherosclerosis Research.* 4: 239, 1964.

———. Atherosclerosis in the Masai. *American Journal of Epidemiology.* 95: 26–37, 1972.

Maurer, B. J., M.D. Changes in grafted and non-grafted coronary arteries, following saphenous vein bypass grafting. *Circulation.* 50: 293, 1974.

Mazess, Richard B., M.D. Bone mineral content of North Alaskan Eskimos. *American Journal of Clinical Nutrition.* 27: 916–925, 1974.

McCarron, David A., M.D. Blood pressure nutrient intake in the United States. *Science Magazine.* 224: 1392–1398, June 1984.

McIntosh, H. D., M.D., and Jorge A. Garcia, M.D. The first decade of aortocoronary bypass grafting, 1967–1977. Special article, a review. *Circulation.* 57: 405–431, 1978.

Menzen, Daniel, M.D. Vitamin E found to protect mouse lung in polluted air. *Medical Tribune.* May 3, 1978.

Mertz, W., M.D. Effects and metabolism of glucose tolerance factor. *Nutrition Review.* 33: 1929, 1975.

Mitch, William E., M.D., et al. The effect of a keto acid–amino acid supplement to a restricted diet on the progression of chronic renal failure. *New England Journal of Medicine.* 311: 623–629, 1984.

Morris, J. N. Coronary heart disease and physical activity of work. *The Lancet.* 2:1053, 111 (November 21 and November 28), 1953.

———. Vigorous exercise in leisure time in the incidence of coronary heart-disease. *The Lancet.* 1:333–339, 1973.

Mundth, E. D., M.D. Surgical measures for coronary heart disease. *New England Journal of Medicine.* 293: 13, 75, 124, 1975.

Murphy, Marvin L., M.D., et al. Treatment of chronic stable angina; a preliminary report of survival data of the randomized Veterans Administration Cooperative study. *New England Journal of Medicine.* 297: 621–627, 1977.

Newman, H. I., M.D. Serum chromium and angiographically determined coronary artery disease. *Clinical Chemistries.* 24: 541, 1978.

Newmark, H. L., M.D. Stability of B_{12} in the presence of ascorbic acid. *American Journal of Clinical Nutrition.* 29: 645–649, 1976.

Norum, Kaare, M.D. Some present concepts concerning diet and prevention of coronary heart disease. *Nutrition and Metabolism.* 22: 1–7, 1978.

Olson, Robert E. The effects of dietary protein, fat, and choline upon the serum lipids and lipoproteins of the rat. *American Journal of Clinical Nutrition.* 6: 111–118, 1958.

Olthof, H., M.D. The definition of myocardial infarction during aortocoronary bypass surgery. *American Heart Journal.* 106: 631–637, Oct. 1983.

Orenstein, Jan Marc, M.D., Ph.D. Micro emboli observed in deaths following coronary pulmonary bypass surgery: Silicone antifoam agents and polyvinyl chloride tubing as source of emboli. *Human Pathology.* 13: 1082–1090, 1982.

Ornish, Dean, M.D., et al. Effects of stress management training and dietary changes in treating ischemic heart disease. *Journal of the American Medical Association.* 249: 54–59, 1983.

Orr, William C., Ph.D. Sleep disturbances after open heart surgery. *American Journal of Cardiology.* 39: 196, 1977.

Öst, C. R., M.D. Regression of peripheral atherosclerosis during therapy with high doses of nicotenic acid. *Scandinavian Journal of Clinical and Laboratory Investigation.* Supplement 93: 241–245, 1967.

Paffenbarger, R. S., M.D. Work energy level: Personal characteristics and fatal heart attack, a birth cohort effect. *American Journal of Epidemiology.* 105: 200–213, 1977.

Peters, Ruth K., D.Sc. Physical fitness in subsequent myocardial infarction in healthy workers. *Journal of the American Medical Association.* 240: 3052–3056, 1983.

Podrid, Philip J., M.D., et al. Prognosis of medically treated patients with coronary artery disease with profound ST segment depression during exercise testing. *New England Journal of Medicine.* 305: 1111–1116, Nov. 1981.

Price, D. L., M.D. Cholesterol emboli and cerebral arteries as a complication of retrograde aortic profusion during cardiac surgery. *Neurology.* 20: 1209–1214, 1970.

Puska, Pekka, M.D. Controlled, randomised trial of the effect of dietary fat on blood pressure. *The Lancet.* 1: Jan. 8, 1983.

Regan, Timothy, M.D. Myocardial blood flow and oxygen consumption during postprandial lipemia and heparin-induced lipolyse. *Circulation.* 23: 55–63, 1961.

Rimm, A. A., M.D. Changes in occupation after aorta coronary bypass operation. *Journal of the American Medical Association.* 236: 361, 1976.

Ross, Richard S., M.D. Lewis A. Connor memorial lecture: The next 30 years—will the progress continue? *Circulation.* 62: 1–7, 1980.

Roth, D., M.D. Non-invasive and invasive demonstration of spontaneous regression of coronary artery disease. *Circulation.* 62, 888–896, 1980.

Rouse, Ian L., M.D. Blood pressure—lowering effect of a vegetarian diet: control, trial and normal tensive subjects. *The Lancet.* 1: 5–9, Jan. 1983.

Russell, Richard O., M.D. Symptomatic patient after coronary bypass surgery. *Primary Cardiology.* 14–25, June 1983.

Sacks, Frank M., M.D. Blood pressure in vegetarians. *American Journal of Epidemiology.* 100: 390–398.

———. Effect of ingestion of meat on plasma cholesterol of vegetarians. *Journal of the American Medical Association.* 246: 640–644, 1981.

———. Ingestion of egg raises plasma low density lipoprotein in free living subjects. *The Lancet.* 647–649, March 24, 1984.

Savageau, J. A. Neuropsychological dysfunction following elective cardiac operation. *Journal of Thoracic Cardiovascular Surgery.* 84: 585–594, 1982.

Schroeder, Henry A., M.D. Chromium deficiency as a factor in atherosclerosis. *Journal of Chronic Diseases.* 23: 123–142, 1970.

Schulze, E. Zeber das verhalten des cholesterins gegen das licht. *Z. Physiol. Chem.* 43: 316, 1904.

Seides, Stuart, F., M.D. Coronary problems after bypass surgery. *New England Journal of Medicine.* 298: 1213–1217, 1978.

Shekelle, Richard B., Ph.D. Diet, serum cholesterol, and death from coronary heart disease. Western Electric Study. *New England Journal of Medicine.* 304: 65–70, 1981.

Sherman, H. C., M.D. Calcium requirement in man. *Journal of Biological Chemistry.* 44: 21, 1920.

Slogoff, S., M.D. Ediologic factors in neuropsychiatric complications association with cardiopulmonary bypass. *Anesthesia and Analgesia.* 61: 903–911, 1982.

Soloff, L. A., M.D. Cardiac deterioration replacing cardiac pain after surgery to revascularize the heart. *American Heart Journal.* 84: 446, 1972.

Spittle, C. R., M.D. Atherosclerosis and Vitamin C. *The Lancet.* 2: 1280, 1971.

Strom, A., M.D. Examination of the diet of Norwegian families during the war years, 1942–1944. *Active Medicus Scandinavia.* Supplement 214: 47, 1948.

———. Mortality from circulatory diseases in Norway. *The Lancet.* 126–129, 1951.

Taylor, K. M., M.D. Brain damage during open heart surgery. An editorial. *Thorax.* 37: 873–876, 1982.

ter Welle, H. F., M.D. The effect of soya lecithin on serum lipid values in type 2, hyperlipoproteinemia. *Activ. Med. Scandinavia.* 195: 267–271, 1974.

Vartiainen, Ilmari, M.D. Wartime immortality of certain diseases in Finland. *Annals of Internal Medicine,* Finland. 535: 234–240, 1946.

———, and K. Kanerva, M.D. Arteriosclerosis in wartime. *Annals of Internal Medicine,* Finland. 536: 748–758, 1947.

Vesselinovitch, D., M.D. Studies of reversal of advanced atherosclerosis in rhesus monkeys. *American Journal of Pathology.* 70: 41A, 1973.

———. Regression of atherosclerosis in rabbits, treatment with low fat diet, hyperoxia, and hypolipidemic agents. *Atherosclerosis.* 19: 259–275, 1974.

The Veterans Administration Coronary Artery Bypass Surgery Cooperative Study Group. Eleven-year survival in the Veterans Administration randomized trial of coronary bypass surgery for stable angina. *New England Journal of Medicine.* 311: 1333–1339, 1984.

Walker, Ruth M., M.D. Calcium retention in the adult human male, as effective by protein intake. *Journal of Nutrition.* 102: 1297–1302, 1972.

Whelton, P. K., M.D. New trial tightens link between thiazides and cardiac arrythmia. *Medical World News.* 32: Jan. 24, 1983.

Whitaker, Julian M., M.D. A natural approach to heart disease, a review. *Journal of Applied Nutrition.* 34: 103–110, 1982.

Williams, A. V., M.D. Increased blood cell agglutination following ingestion of fat, a factor contributing to cardiac ischemia, coronary insufficiency, and anginal pain. *Angiology.* 8: 29, 1957.

Williams, Roger J., M.D. Concept of genetotrophic disease. *Nutrition Review.* 8: 257–260, 1950.

Willis, G. C., M.D. The reversibility of atherosclerosis. *Canadian Medical Association Journal.* 77: 106, 1957.

Wissler, Robert W., M.D. Studies of progression of advanced atherosclerosis in experimental animals and man. *Annals of New York Academy of Science.* 275: 363–378, 1976.

———. Regression of atherosclerosis in experimental animals and man. *Modern Concepts of Cardiovascular Disease.* 46: 27–32, 1977.

World Health Organization Technical Report. Series No. 522. Energy and protein requirements. Geneva, 1973.

Wright, Irving S., M.D. Correct levels of serum cholesterol, average versus normal versus optimal. *Journal of the American Medical Association.* 236: 261–262, 1976.

Index